Dr. Duke's
Essential Herbs

Dr. Duke's Essential Herbs

13 VITAL HERBS YOU NEED TO
- Disease-proof your body
- Boost your energy
- Lengthen your life

James A. Duke, Ph.D.

RODALE
REACH™

An Imprint of Rodale Books

Notice

This book is meant to increase your knowledge of the latest developments in the use of plants for medicinal purposes. Because everyone is different, a physician must diagnose conditions and supervise the use of healing herbs to treat individual health problems. Herbs and other natural remedies are not substitutes for professional medical care. We urge you to seek the best medical resources available to help you make informed decisions.

Cover Designers: Andrew Newman, Carol Angstadt
Cover Photographer: Anthony Loew
Interior Designer: Faith Hague
Illustrator: Peggy K. Duke

ISBN 1–57954–183–6 hardcover

Distributed to the book trade by St. Martin's Press

2 4 6 8 10 9 7 5 3 1 hardcover

Visit us on the Web at www.rodalebooks.com, or call us toll-free at (800) 848-4735.

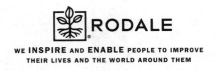

RODALE

WE INSPIRE AND ENABLE PEOPLE TO IMPROVE
THEIR LIVES AND THE WORLD AROUND THEM

This book is dedicated to our adventurous ancestors, yours
and mine, who learned through hard experience and over the
course of many millennia which plants were edible, which were
medicinal, and which were poisonous. They passed down their
genes to us, so that our genes recognize and utilize many of
these natural substances as nutrients and medicines.

Contents

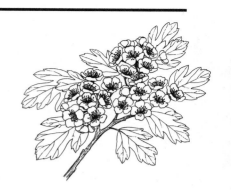

Acknowledgments

To Mom and Dad, for handing down the genes that enabled me to survive long enough to write this book and, in turn, help a few more people to survive a little longer, too.

To my many right hands: Judi DuCellier, Mary Jo Bogenshutz-Godwin, Peggy Duke, Leigh Broadhurst, Stephen Beckstrom Sternberg, Kerrie Kyde, and Ellen Gordon. Each of them contributed a lot of nice things to this book, often without even knowing it.

To the patient team of writers who worked faithfully to translate my jargon into layman's terms. They had a challenging and thankless job. During the course of writing this book, they tracked me down in all sorts of interesting places: Australia, California, Utah, and Washington State, not to mention home-sweet-home. They found me, and they challenged me, and for that, I thank them. Challenge is a two-way street and good for all involved.

To my editors at Rodale, who willingly put up with a cantankerous, overcommitted, 70-year-old reprobate.

chapter one

Herbs for Good Health

First the word, then the plant, lastly the knife.
—Aesculapius of Thassaly, Greek god of healing, circa 1200 B.C.

BY THE TIME THEY REACH THEIR SEVENTIES, most people take seven different synthetic medications every day. All last year, I took only seven. (They were all over-the-counter Aleve tablets for my arthritic knee.)

I think I've chanced upon a better way to maintain health, a way that's much better than the prescription drug path.

Chalk up much of my good fortune to good genes, good diet, good exercise, good stress management, and a measure of good luck. The rest of it, I'm firmly convinced, stems from ingesting herbs and herbal supplements.

Will herbs and their phytomedicines improve *your* health and reverse illness? Should you bother to read this entire book to find out? Follow along with my "Five Ifs," and you'll know right away.

If you can afford to go to your doctor and pay for all the medications he or she prescribes

If you can communicate with your physician comfortably and have faith in him or her

If your doctor correctly diagnoses your ailments

If you have one and only one health problem

If you know beyond a shadow of a doubt that you're not defi-cient in a vitamin, mineral, amino acid, essential fatty acid, or any other nutrient

. . . then put this book back on the shelf. You don't need it and couldn't appreciate the advice contained herein. Your doctor's man-made magic silver bullet may actually help you. It really may be one of the best possible medicines for you.

Iffy Propositions

Still with me? Thought so.

I can be so seemingly brazen because few people can answer each of these five ifs positively. Let's fill in a little detail behind each of these conditions.

Means. More than 10 percent of all Americans can't afford to go to a doctor or pay for a prescription. Across the world, 80 percent of all people lack such financial means. Some 43 million Americans, as of July 1999, have no health insurance. (For more information, see "Cheaper by the Duke's Dozen" on page 4.)

Communication. The average HMO doctor spends about six minutes with each patient. He or she probably spends more time making a sandwich during a commercial break.

I was shocked when I heard the following sorry statistic, from none other than former Surgeon General C. Everett Koop, M.D., who spoke at the World Med Conference in the Greater Washington Met-ropolitan Area in 1996. After asking a question, male physicians in-terrupt a patient's answer in an average of 14 seconds. Female physicians are somewhat more polite, interrupting rambling patients after about 40 seconds. No wonder surveys report that most people feel they can't communicate effectively with doctors.

Accuracy. In detecting Lyme disease, physician's diagnoses are wrong 50 percent of the time. They bat somewhat better or worse with other ailments. Twenty percent of all hacking done at doctors' offices are undiagnosed cases of whooping cough (pertussis), according to a 1996 issue of *Science News*.

Sickness. Few of us have one and only one ailment at any given time. Whether we (or our doctors) know it or not, several things are usually wrong.

Nourishment. We all like to eat, and we all think we eat rather healthfully. But no matter how well-fed you might be, there's a good chance you don't ingest optimum amounts of many nutrients. A lot of us are deficient in basic vitamins and minerals.

In contrast to the pharmaceutical industry's perfect poster person, I offer you myself: Though I still can afford my doctor and my doctor's prescriptions, I try not to buy into the deal. I talk quite plainly and am easy to understand. I'm never presumptuous enough to diagnose, but I can make guesses and take wild stabs that are sometimes correct. I have a handful of health concerns of my own for which I'd like answers. And while I can chow down with the best of them, I still don't think I or anyone else can consume sufficient amounts of some fundamental nutrients solely from food. I've learned enough in my day as a botanist to know that the vegetables, fruits, and plants we eat often are almost bereft of nutrition (especially given how breeders and the food industry process them).

What's *Really* Safe?

Every once in a while, you'll hear a story on the evening news about someone dying from an extreme allergic reaction to something he or she has eaten. In 1998, about 100 people died in the United States after ingesting common, ordinary nuts. In the same period, fewer than 100 Americans died after consuming an herb in some form, and more than 90 percent of these people were intentionally abusing certain of the more potent members of our herbal pharmacy. To the best of my knowledge, no one died in the United States in 1998 from ingesting an herbal product in a safe, recommended dosage.

Yet critics of phytomedicine cite safety as a primary concern. The faultfinders apparently want zero jeopardy and absolute safety from herbs. I guess we can therefore expect that from their preferred medicines, synthetic drugs, right? Hardly. Once those things ricochet around inside the body, they kill by the thousands.

In 1994, between 70,000 and 130,000 people in the United States died because of the pharmaceuticals they took—pharmaceuticals that were properly prescribed and duly taken. It has been implicated that, every year, complications from taking commonplace nonsteroidal anti-inflammatory drugs (NSAIDs) cause about 7,600 deaths.

Of all people admitted to the hospital, 30 percent will suffer an adverse effect to a properly prescribed drug, according to the Boston Collaborative Drug Surveillance Project. Anywhere from 3 to 28 percent of all hospital admissions are related to a bad reaction to a medication. In other words, bad reactions to medications will kill 3 out of every 1,000 people who go to a hospital, according to a 1997 report in the *Journal of the American Medical Association*.

Cheaper by the Duke's Dozen

Here's a cost comparison between leading synthetic pharmaceuticals and the equivalent phytomedicinal dosage.

Condition	Pharmaceutical	Herbal
Alzheimer's disease	Cognex $5.63	Ginkgo biloba $.59
Angina, cardiopathy	Verapamil $.51	Hawthorn $.37
Anxiety, stress	Valium $2.15	Kava kava $1.18
Arthritis	Hydrocortisone $2.78	Turmeric $.77
Benign prostate enlargement	Proscar $2.86 Hytrin $1.55	Saw palmetto $.98 Evening primrose $.59
Chronic venous insufficiency	Compress or stockings $2.78	Horse chestnut $.29
Cirrhosis, hepatosis	Interferon $120.49	Milk thistle $2.16
Depression	Zoloft $2.25	St. John's wort $.50
Flu, bronchitis, colds	Flumadine $4.98	Echinacea $1.60
Gout	Allopurinol $.70	Celery seed extract $.60
High cholesterol	Zocor $3.73	Garlic $.23
Maculitis	Eyeglasses $200	Bilberry $1.07

Let us not forget the emotional toll exacted on thousands and thousands of families that lose a loved one in the blink of an eye simply because that poor person followed doctor's orders and took some synthetic substance.

True, few, if any, herbal supplements have been proven safe and effective—at least not in strictly conducted American studies. But average people have been conducting their own informal studies on herbs for millennia, and we get fewer than 100 deaths a year, primarily from ill-advised, intentional overdosing. In ironic contrast, ostensibly above-average scientists have been conducting rigidly controlled experiments on synthetic medications and making exacting calculations for the last several decades, and we get thousands and thousands of deaths.

Let the Best (Medicine) Man Win

As early as a decade ago, more North Americans went to alternative or unconventional practitioners than to orthodox, by-the-book primary-care physicians (an estimated 425 million visits, compared with 386 million). People spent about $13.7 billion on unconventional therapies back in 1990, most of it ($10.3 billion) unreimbursed by an HMO, according to a 1993 report in the *New England Journal of Medicine*.

And the numbers are rising. People wouldn't continue with alternative therapies if they didn't like the service they received or they weren't helped. Perhaps they're not being harmed quite so much. At the very least, I believe, one explanation is a more comfortable experience. Usually, alternative practitioners are more laid-back. They understand the deleterious impact of stress, and they're not going to look over a shoulder nervously at the clock, wondering what their bosses are going to think about the bottom line if they spend too much time with you. They're not impatient with patients. They take the time to listen to you and answer your questions.

But service with a smile doesn't completely explain why people are drawn to alternative practitioners and herbal medicines. The better reason is, simply, that herbal medications work. I see proof every day. I hear about it all the time from colleagues. And I read about it in medical journal studies, many of them done in Europe and Japan, where the bulk of the herbal research is being conducted. In the rest of the world, herbs are regarded as the rivals they truly are to prescription drugs.

In Germany, for instance, physicians and pharmacists are required to study herbal medicine in school as a condition to get a license. General practitioners, especially, routinely prescribe natural, plant-based medications. The German government has also established a panel of experts, called Commission E, that has evaluated more than 300 medicinal plants specifically to give doctors and consumers therapeutic guidance in how to safely and most effectively use herbs. The entire collection of reviews has been translated into English by the American Botanical Council and gathered into a book. *The German Commission E Monographs*, as it's called, has quickly become a standard reference for what herbs to take and how.

Why are natural plant chemicals worthy pharmaceutical rivals? Because they often work on the same physiologic pathways and principles as their prescription counterparts. The big difference is that phytochemicals work along several circuits simultaneously and naturally. The pharmaceutical usually is a single substance that works on one circuit or two. I think of it as the difference between a shotgun and a bullet. The magic bullet is precision-targeted and has no regard for how it might disrupt the rest of the body. Herbs are shotgun blasts that contain thousands of natural active phytochemicals—some that will help with the correctly diagnosed ailment, others that will help with undiagnosed and unknown problems, and still others that are just plain good for you that you probably need anyway. If you don't need them, your body still will make good use of them.

Everyone into the (Gene) Pool!

You might look like a person, but you're actually just a big jar of genes, those strands of DNA and RNA (ribonucleic acid) that determine the traits and functions of proteins and other genetic material. Like viruses and bacteria, your 100,000 or so genes are always trying to reproduce themselves. Over the ages, they've seen just about everything, and they always attempt to maintain a good equilibrium, which includes good health. Disease, on the other hand, upsets the apple cart, introducing a disequilibrium.

Your ancestors—not just your great-grandparents or even your great-great-great-grandparents, but your distant evolutionary relatives—grew up and evolved with thousands of phytochemicals. (What's a phytochemical? The prefix *phyto-* simply means "plant-based," so a phytochemical is any chemical or substance that comes from a plant. Phytomedicine is medical care based on plant therapy.) Your kin and mine, distant and near, consumed these natural compounds and survived on them, learning by trial and error what was edible, what was poisonous, and what fell into the intermediate category we now describe as medicinal. In ways we can hardly fathom, they passed on to you and me genes that are familiar with these chemicals. As far as we know, our genes may be utterly dependent on some of these substances. Your chromosomes might be crying out for some of them that your diet no longer provides.

You and I, in other words, evolved with these disease-preventing, illness-treating foods and phytomedicines. We didn't evolve with synthetic drugs. Our genes encountered synthetics for the very first time fewer than 200 years ago.

It's Not Nice to Rule Mother Nature

Even with a semi-synthetic medicinal monstrosity that's partly based on a natural compound, our genes aren't likely to get a deja-vu sense of vague familiarity and friendliness. Trust me, plants have been around a long time, and many, many mutations have come and gone. I'll bet that evolution and mere chance have already tried most of the chemical variations that medical science has tried or could possibly try. If such variations (mutations) aided plant survival in the grand evolutionary scheme of things, the modification would have remained. If not, the plant or its offspring didn't thrive and may have died, along with the mutation.

But science, hell-bent on improving upon Mother Nature and trying to reinvent her already discarded misshapen wheels, keeps tinkering with phytochemicals. I could give many examples, but I'll relate an anecdote about the mayapple.

As a treatment for venereal warts and other viral disorders, the mayapple has a long history in both folk medicine and real medicine. But only in 1984 was its medicinal value affirmed with the approval of a mayapple-derived drug (etoposide) for testicular cancer.

Research had uncovered four chemicals, called lignans, in the mayapple's rhizome, the underground stem that a non-botanist would call the root, that proved to work synergistically against the herpes virus. Not content to leave well enough alone, some scientist in some lab got the bright idea to chemically alter one of the lignans. I'll wager that in the last several thousand years, evolution already tried and ditched that very same alteration.

I don't really think the change made the resulting new compound any better or, at least as far as we know right now, any worse. But it for sure made it proprietary. And that meant it could be patented. The patented substance has since sold for more than a billion dollars, often as high as $400 million per year.

It's difficult to patent a natural phytochemical, because Mother Nature already holds the patent on it. And you can't make much of a profit unless *you* hold the patent. By modifying, for better or worse, a natural compound, you can obtain a patent much more easily. The industry's driving force, in other words, is not so much human health and well-being as it is corporate patentability and profitability.

Hissing in the Wind

In the last decade or so, hardly a day has gone by without news of another marvel of nutritional medicine. The evidence is so overwhelming at this point that it's beyond dispute. It wasn't that long ago, though, that medical journals and so-called quackbusters, those self-styled guardians of public welfare, proclaimed that vitamins enriched only your urine and the bank accounts of the supplement makers. But at the same time they denounced nutrient supplements, fans of pharmaceuticals were buying up supplement companies, and more and more physicians started taking the very vitamins and minerals that they wouldn't prescribe to their patients. Did the drug firms and the doctors know something that they didn't admit?

An analogous situation exists today. A few die-hards out there still denounce vitamins, minerals, and other nutrients, but they and their protégés have shifted focus, taking aim at herbs and loudly telling us that medicinal plants are dangerous, useless, unproven folk-lore, wives' tales, and witches' brews that certainly won't help and might hurt. At the same time, pharmaceutical giants are gobbling up herb manufacturers and trying to isolate and patent certain active ingredients (magic silver bullets).

We're not trying to kill vampires and werewolves here. We don't need silver bullets. The gentler phytomedicinal doses from herbal supplements, even herbs grown in your backyard, are the crowning achievement of thousands upon thousands of years of research and testing. They're efficacious. They're safe. I've dedicated the rest of my life to compelling American medicine to fairly compare its drugs to nature's and acknowledge this truth.

Duke's Dozen for Better Health

Without further adieu, here is Duke's Dozen—a baker's dozen, given that I've chosen 13. These herbs are the ones that I'm most likely to take day to day, the ones that many, if not most, people will find improve their health.

Bilberry. Whatever reason you have for sore eyes, this blueberry relative is quite a sight. I don't understand how carrots stole the lime-light from this plant's tiny round fruits, which contain mighty antioxidants that have long been associated with averting vision disorders, including macular degeneration, retinopathy, and retinitis. They also may deter cataracts and glaucoma.

Celery and celery seed. This is my main mandatory medicinal plant, the only one (besides coffee, also a medicinal plant) that I take every day of the year. For more than three years, celery has kept me free of my one big health problem: gout. Though big in Australia, few others have acknowledged celery's ability to prevent this most debilitating joint pain. As long as I take my celery seed extract, I no longer need the antigout medications that I depended on for most of two decades.

Echinacea. Echinacea is the herbal equivalent of vitamin C. To Plains Indians, echinacea was a cure-all. They, along with many other Americans up through the nineteenth century, used it for just about every health problem that cropped up. They were probably right to do so. Science now documents that the purple coneflower, as it's also known, enhances the immune system, fights viruses, and kills bacteria. Whether you have a cold, a sore throat, the flu, bronchitis, or anything in between, you want echinacea. The American medical establishment says echinacea won't prevent colds or the flu. The American medical establishment, I think, is wrong.

Auntie, Get Your Oxidant

Antioxidants are among phytomedicine's star attractions. They do for biological cells what a good coat of Rustoleum does for an iron gate: prevent a destructive molecular reaction with the very air we breathe.

Oxygen is essential for us to live, needless to say, but in return for allowing us to inhale, exhale, and generate energy, it triggers a rather nasty side effect. In a byproduct of the molecular reaction, it forms molecularly unstable molecules, called free radicals, that are able to go out on a search-and-destroy mission that can kill other cells.

A free radical does what it does because it lacks an electron. It's hell-bent on getting one, too, and it knows no bounds in striking out to get what it wants. It'll attack any molecule it chances upon. In the process of stealing the electron, it often transforms its victim into a free-radical molecule, perpetuating a vicious chain reaction.

Oxidation is why food spoils, why butter gets rancid, why that log in your fireplace burns so warmly, and, partly, why people get old, go blind, get cholesterol blockages in their arteries, or get age spots on their skin. The same reaction that allows a fresh coat of paint to dry or makes a banana turn brown is also at work inside and outside of your body. The only difference, essentially, is which molecules are assaulted.

Evening primrose. In Europe, this night-blooming plant is a favored ornamental flower and a favored medicinal plant. In the United States, most people dismiss it as a weed. The discrepancy in perspective sort of sums up the difference in mindset on either side of the Atlantic regarding herbal medicine.

Oil of evening primrose is one of our best sources of gamma-linolenic acid (GLA), an essential omega-6 fatty acid sorely lacking in the average person's diet. Without GLA, our bodies couldn't manufacture prostaglandins, highly therapeutic compounds responsible for, to name just a few functions, controlling abnormal cell growth; relaxing blood vessels; balancing the immune, glandular, and nervous systems; regulating body temperature; and metabolizing cholesterol.

For women, evening primrose brings relief from nagging pre-

Over the last several eons, nature figured out a way to cope with the inevitability of oxidation. It came up with antioxidants. The mechanism differs from antioxidant to antioxidant, but the outcome always remains the same: These selfless natural substances sacrifice themselves readily so that other molecules may escape unscathed. Antioxidants appear in every green leaf out there, protecting them from damage by the very oxygen they produce. And what they do for plants they can do for people: avert entirely, mitigate, or at least slow down a lot of harmful processes, including diseases and aging.

Vitamin C, vitamin E, and beta-carotene are among the better-known antioxidants in the nutritional world. By no means do I mean to downplay their medicinal value, for they help prevent health problems in ways no other antioxidants can. But they're just a trio of fish in a sea of other phytochemical antioxidants that also possess unique abilities. Bilberry, for instance, favors the blood vessels and tissues in your eyes. Turmeric, on the other hand, is better at protecting your joints.

Just one or two won't cut it, health-wise. You need a wide sampling of nature's antioxidant power.

menstrual nuisances. For me and a lot of other older men, it contributes to a healthier prostate gland. Regardless of gender, the plant's oils promise to retard the nerve deterioration so often seen in diabetes, the skin inflammation of eczema, the bronchial restriction in asthma, and the head-hammering pain of a migraine. The herb also provides the antioxidant bioflavonoid quercetin, which helps your heart, and the amino acid L-tryptophan, a natural antidepressant and sedative.

Garlic. Based on personal experience, I can attest that these pungent cloves do indeed ward off vampire bats (and, presumably, vampires). But the herb also keeps away more imminent threats, such as high blood pressure, high cholesterol, bacteria, and viruses.

I take garlic as an echinacea adjunct, because it, too, bolsters the immune system. To me, it's nature's version of synthetic penicillin. Many other people will want the cardiovascular protection it confers without the serious consequences its pharmaceutical rivals impose. Or perhaps you might benefit best from its ability to help your liver dispose of toxins.

Ginkgo. Good health has kept me in circulation all over the globe, and ginkgo biloba, of late, has been helping to keep my blood in circulation. The concentrated extract from this tree's leaves improves blood flow from your brain to your feet, plus strategic points in between.

Poor circulation is a hallmark of aging. Better blood flow helps to maintain sharper mental function, deterring Alzheimer's disease and other types of age-related mental decline. It prevents the heart from working unnecessarily hard and preserves feeling and dexterity in the hands and feet. It even helps sustain sexual function in the genitalia. Studies, you'll learn, show that ginkgo extracts work just as well as some anticoagulant and anti-Alzheimer's drugs.

Hawthorn. Virtually complete cardiac care comes in this crab apple–like container. The phytochemicals in hawthorn berries address almost every facet of heart disease. They help stabilize heart rhythm, maintain good blood pressure, keep arteries clear of blockages and allow blood to circulate fully, fight high cholesterol, minimize chest pains, counteract fluid retention and tissue swelling, and avert shortness of breath.

In case the doctors out there don't understand plain English, I'll rephrase in more pharmaceutical terms: Hawthorn provides the ABC's and even the D of mainstream cardiac care. Top this, if you can:

A. Angiotensin-converting enzyme inhibitors

B. Beta-blockers

C. Calcium-channel blockers

D. Diuretics

I once smoked like a chimney, and though I've long since given up cigarettes, I'm sure some cardiovascular damage has been done. I also still regularly put myself through an insanely taxing schedule. Stress and cigarette smoking are both major contributors to heart disease, and that's why hawthorn is one of my most trusted herbs.

Horse chestnut. At the age of 70, you'd think I'd be the perfect candidate for varicose veins. But I'm not. Varicose verse, perhaps, (as you'll see in "The Key to the Medicine Cabinet" on page 14) but not varicose veins.

Sure, spider veins creep down my legs, but they haven't transformed into varicose veins or, worse, a condition called chronic venous insufficiency, in which blood vessels starving for blood swell up and cause aches or cramping in your legs. "Neigh"-sayers may assert otherwise, but I think horse chestnut is responsible. The same chemicals in the plant that ease inflammation and facilitate leg circulation do the same for the swollen rectal veins responsible for hemorrhoids.

Kava kava. What coffee is to waking up, kava is to calming down. It's the ideal antidote to an always-on-the-go, stress-filled lifestyle; it's the natural substitute for Valium and similar pharmaceutical sedatives and tranquilizers.

Whether or not you enjoy caffeine as a pick-me-up, you'll probably like kava as a tranquil put-me-down. If you're agitated by anxiety or can't fall asleep at night, kava can smooth your furrowed brow. It also can be a reliable alternative to drugs for some hyperactive children.

Milk thistle. If you wet your whistle, better stock up on milk thistle. It's too easy to call this lovely plant a boozer's best friend. You don't need to have cirrhosis, and you don't need to overindulge in too much of the rye, the corn, or the grape. Anyone concerned about the health of his or her liver, whether because of hepatitis, exposure to

(continued on page 16)

The Key to the Medicine Cabinet

If I couldn't play the guitar, I might not have learned as much as I've learned about nature's pharmacy. Plants have been close friends for 65 years. The guitar has been a close friend for all but five of those years.

Music, the old quote goes, hath charms to soothe the savage breast (or beast). But that's hardly the extent of its allure. For me, it's been the key that opened doors to some amazing ethnobotanical secrets.

How could a 16-year-old North Carolina redneck who played bass fiddle with Homer A. Briarhopper and the Dixie Dudes ever have expected that his music could become an ethnobotanical tool? Sure, I couldn't have spent so many years as a specialist in medicinal plants at the U.S. Department of Agriculture Research Station in Beltsville, Maryland, without a degree in botany. But my finger-picking background (I was originally a music major, and it helped me pay my way through college) opened the doors, hearts, and mouths of a lot of native Latin Americans who otherwise would've been suspicious and tight-lipped. I travel widely in the Southern Hemisphere in search of new species of medicinal plants, and I doubt that I could've made the inroads and friendships throughout the Amazon necessary to discover the mysteries of local therapeutic herbs.

Even after I acquired a fluency in local Spanish dialects, music was a common language. With an acoustic guitar on my back or in my lap and a corny song in my heart, I've been welcomed with astounding heart-warming hospitality almost everywhere I've ventured in the jungles. As an ice-breaker and an inducement to being brought into the inner circles of local medicine, a guitar turns out to be better (not to mention far healthier) than packs of cigarettes and cases of rum.

I can't count the number of times I've been on excursions with incompatible people from drastically divergent cultures who end up being the best of pals because of music. Typically, we spend all day trudging through hot jungles, sloshing through interminable waist-high swamps and fording crocodile-infested backwaters. We live and sleep together in close quarters with no electricity, no amenities—not much more than rice and beans with hot peppers cooked over an open fire. Yet with a guitar or two on hand, people who have been at each other's throats a few hours before are singing in harmony and reaching only to wrap their arms around their newfound buddies' shoulders.

Music is also particularly important to the shamans, the indigenous medicine men and women of the Amazon and other third-world forest areas. My own shaman and healer in Peru, Don Antonio Montero Pisco, has a song for each of dozens of medicinal herbs and the treatments with which he uses them. When I took some of my retirement income five years ago and established the ReNuPeru Garden, a five-acre parcel in Peru that's part of the nonprofit Amazon Center for Environmental Education and Research (ACEER), I stipulated that Don Antonio be hired to create and oversee the garden. I knew he'd be able to develop the land, bring in important medicinal species, and teach both the local population and visitors how to cultivate and use them. Through his work, which I help to sustain with a small annual donation and an ongoing search for matching funds, entire villages will be able to keep themselves healthy for a long time.

Don Antonio understands music. He's got an intuitive sense of notes, chords, scales, and rhythm that he demonstrates in each song he sings as a paean to each herb. I've tried to learn from him. I think I have. He at least influenced some of the music I play. I, too, sing praise to nature's medicines and pen poems in homage to them. But while Don Antonio is more like the Amazon's answer to Amadeus, I'm afraid I'm more like the Spike Jones of ginseng, the Groucho of ginkgo, the Jerry Lewis of limericks, or the McCartney of the mayapple.

No, I've never penned a song with lyrics that read, When I find myself in deep, deep trouble/Mother Nature comes to me/Bringing Duke's Dozen/Bilber-ry to cel-e-ry. But some of the lyrics are almost as bad. I call them my Varicose Verse. As I tour the United States and the world and lecture on herbal medicine, people have come to expect (or dread) a song or two before I conclude a talk. Nature's Herbs even distributes copies of my CD HerbAlbum to those with the temerity to give it a listen.

To be serious for a second: Music means more to me than words adequately describe. It's a constant companion, a source of solace, fun, inspiration, and sentimentality. At the party for my 70th birthday in April 1999, my son John made me cry when, as I played my instrumental version of "Sunday Morning Sidewalk," he walked in, picked up a guitar, and started to accompany me, augmenting my playing with his own licks. He jerked another tear out of my eyes with his rendition of Hank Williams Jr.'s "Old Habits are Hard to Break." The song led him to open up to me for the first time about how much he enjoyed his formative years here at the vineyard and even back when we boated on the Rio Pirre in Panama.

Another song, another unlocked door, another treasure trove of secrets.

suspected toxins, or any other reason, can benefit from milk thistle supplements.

Silymarin, one of the medicinal compounds in the plant, both strengthens the outer surface of the liver, which helps to discourage toxic chemicals from getting through, and encourages an enzymatic action that spurs better cellular regeneration, which allows the organ to detoxify the bloodstream more efficiently.

St. John's wort. When days grow short and nights turn cold, I become depressed, listless, and SAD (the acronym for seasonal affective disorder) unless this supplemental patron saint of mental serenity is with me. St. John's is almost like sunshine in a bottle. If I can't go to a place like the Amazon with 12 hours of daily equatorial sunshine, I take St. John's wort.

St. John's wort can help relieve a variety of viral problems, from cold sores to chickenpox; its antiviral qualities may even figure into a treatment for HIV infection one day. But this perennial weed works best on the mind, not the body. As most of Europe has long known, St. John's wort is an excellent mood elevator for cases of mild to moderate depression and anxiety—just as effective as its pharmaceutical counterpart, Zoloft (Sertralin). In Germany, supplements outsell Prozac and all other antidepressants combined.

Saw palmetto. The berries on this plant represent one of the best examples of herbal medicine. For relieving problems associated with benign prostate enlargement, a condition that virtually every man will face if he lives long enough, saw palmetto works better than its pharmaceutical equivalent. It goes into action faster, it poses a far smaller risk of side effects, and it works for more men. It's cheaper, too.

You can't ask for more than that, but I'll still do you one better: It may help slow or reverse male pattern baldness, better than its prescription-only rival.

Turmeric. For all those minor aches and pains, most people reach for aspirin or a prescription-strength NSAID. I favor turmeric.

Especially when backed up by ginger and cardamom, its botanical brethren, turmeric gives the NSAID drug cortisone a real run for its money, notably when comparing the risk of side effects and especially in treating such sources of inflammation as tendinitis, bursitis, arthritis, and gout. Turmeric, unlike cortisone and other cortico-steroids, won't raise blood pressure, magnify your risk for osteo-porosis, or make your body tissues suck up water like a sponge.

This quintessential seasoning for all yellow-colored Middle Eastern curry dishes carries a rainbowlike array of anti-inflammato-ries and antioxidants that guard arteries, cells, and cell membranes from damage and, maybe, even from cancer. But that's not all. Cur-cumin and turmeric's other phytochemicals protect your liver against toxins and assist with digestion.

From Womb to Tomb

Each of the 13 herbs addresses a particular problem associated with growing old—and we are all growing old, or at least older. So think of my Duke's Dozen in another sense: Most are for children of all ages.

Disease prevention doesn't start when you near the at-risk age. By no means must you be eligible to draw a Social Security check to benefit from phytomedicines. If you waited until then, it would prob-ably be too late for prevention and you'd need larger doses. If, though, you took these supplements when you were younger, you might not need them as much when retirement time rolls around.

Infants and children. No matter how old you are or what your gender, at a minimum you need antioxidant and anticancer protection. Infants get it from breast milk and then baby foods, many of which contain food-grade phytochemicals. For the littlest ones, I'm quicker to recommend dietary "food farmacy" than medicinal herbs or phy-tochemical extracts. Once beyond the age of two, kids can safely take bilberry, echinacea, evening primrose, milk thistle, turmeric, and garlic (along with its relatives, chives, leeks, and onions). For attention deficit/hyperactivity disorder, some little ones may benefit from kava. (For more information, see "Herbs, Kids, and Risk" on page 18.)

Adults. To the list above, young adults can add celery seed, if they're prone to high blood pressure or gout; St. Johns wort, if they tend to be depressed or compulsive; and saw palmetto, if they're male

(continued on page 20)

Herbs, Kids, and Risk

When I was but a fetus, the choline my mother consumed improved my memory and capacity to learn, according to an article in *Science*. Thanks, Mom. And thanks for predisposing me to enjoy beans, many of which contain decent amounts of this substance, which the body uses to make the brain chemical acetylcholine. A less-than-adequate supply of acetylcholine in the brain has been linked to Alzheimer's disease and cognition difficulties.

Just in 1998, the U.S. Food and Drug Administration finally set a recommended daily allowance (RDA) for choline, a decision that, I hope, will improve the memories and learning potential of countless generations. We can only speculate on how the agency's lack of decisiveness up until then harmed our collective cognitive capabilities.

Choline is a phytochemical like any other. Brazil nuts are loaded with it in the form of lecithin. Dandelion flowers, fava beans, poppy seeds, soybeans, and mung beans also are good lecithin sources, while ginseng, fenugreek leaves, and Chinese angelica (*dong-quai*) contain choline itself.

How, then, can we explain the oft-repeated precautionary notes in the chapters ahead against the use of herbal supplements by pregnant or lactating women? Or the vague warnings that infants and youngsters shouldn't ingest herbs?

Conservatives usually bellow a resounding no! when asked if kids, pregnant women, or breastfeeding mothers should take phytochemicals. Repeatedly throughout the book, I have included cautions to that effect. It is true that there is a marked absence of physician's studies of phytomedicines on these folks. Cautious hesitation is one thing, but all the red flags are quite another. In my mind, the warning or prohibition is mostly one big, fat canard.

I am not a physician. I cannot say that kids, pregnant women, and nursing moms *should* take herbal supplements, and I'm obligated to report the warnings of others ostensibly more schooled than me in such matters. Personally, however, I think the warning is unduly alarmist and inappropriately broad. I'll tell you why here, and I'll tell you what I recommend within my family and circle of friends.

Breastfeed, Best Feed?

Yes, there's a woeful dearth of research on how children, pregnant women, and lactating mothers might react to phytochemicals. (There's a woeful dearth of research on phytochemicals in general.) But the criticism very sneakily implies that pharmaceuticals suffer from no such lack. But they do. The drug giants have done very few studies on how their medications might affect kids, new mothers, and expecting mothers. The need for such research is so great that President Bill Clinton, in 1998, tried to get medicine manufacturers to conduct more pediatric studies. They respectfully declined.

And I very disrespectfully ask how they have any logical justification for criticizing the absence of pediatric studies in phytomedicinal research. In fact, they have less credibility than do the herb advocates. For one thing, they can better afford the half-billion bucks it costs to win FDA approval. For another, we've got competing track records to compare and assess.

Which are you more inclined to trust: something your genes have been familiar with for millions of years or a scientifically proven synthetic chemical that your genes may have never yet encountered? If your child had a cold or an earache, would you feel safer giving him or her a little garlic or a brand-new antibiotic or some other synthetic medicine? If you had that earache or cold while pregnant or lactating, which would you trust more? What about if you had high blood pressure or high cholesterol?

Garlic has rarely been compared scientifically with its pharmaceutical counterparts, so we don't know the better medication. Garlic has side effects; pharmaceuticals have side effects. Garlic has benefits; pharmaceuticals have benefits. Until science sees fit to compare them and determine a winner, we're left to best guesses.

Because I am not a medical doctor, I cannot and will not go on record recommending medications for kids younger than 24 months. But I can tell you what I'd suggest for an infant in the Duke family or for my close friends. With some exceptions and qualifications, I generally would sleep better—and so would the child, I think—knowing that the natural medication was at work. Our genes know the naturals; our genes don't know the pharmaceuticals.

The decision—phytofarmacy or pharmaceutical—should always be made

(continued)

Herbs, Kids, and Risk—Continued

on a case-by-case, illness-by-illness basis, weighing all the merits, hazards, and hoped-for benefits every time. Ideally, I'd also talk everything over with a holistic physician. After sifting through the evidence and arguments, I'd choose the treatment that shows the most promise.

That said, for the most part, I'd rarely be afraid if a child took the very same herbs that I take, whether or not they've reached the ripe old age of two, as long as they ingest pint-size dosages appropriate for their smaller sizes. If my grandkid had an earache, echinacea would be entirely appropriate. If he couldn't sleep, I'd dispense a tiny bit of chamomile. Nausea or seasickness? I'd check to see if I had some peppermint tea. In fact, among my immediate and extended families—and that includes pregnant women and lactating moms as well as infants—I don't hesitate to recommend any one of Duke's Dozen.

Only if the situation were life-threatening might I choose a synthetic over a natural, even taking into account the greater risk of side effects. But even then, I'd have to be certain that the synthetic drug were clearly superior and had a better chance of success.

Nature may have meant for infants to ingest, via breast milk, the same natural medicines that their lactating moms ingest. Breast milk may in fact be a good vehicle for some pediatric medications. Although lactation experts tell me that many medications—synthetic and natural—aren't conveyed from mother to child in signficant amounts, some are, and garlic is one that does get through. Even with the previous caveats in mind, I'd rather that any heir to my herbal vineyard forgo an antibiotic in favor of some garlic-laced breast milk, courtesy of his mom.

and have a family history of male-pattern baldness. If frequently stressed, try kava.

Women may need evening primrose (especially for premenstrual tension), horse chestnut (to deter varicose veins), kava (to help relax), and St. John's wort (to fight the blues).

Saw palmetto is the one male-oriented supplement (although women, you'll read soon, can find use for it, too), and it grows in importance as you grow nearer to that half-century mark.

Days of Time and Doses

In each chapter, I offer specific recommendations for when and how often you should consume a particular herb. Generally, if it's a food or a spice, you can safely eat it every single day of your life (so long as you're not allergic to it). Some other herbs, if they're not foods or spices in standardized supplemental form, shouldn't be consumed for lengthy periods. These more medicinally oriented plants should be saved for specific occasions, such as when you're ill or have a pressing need.

What's what? Of my baker's dozen, these clearly are foods or spices: bilberry, celery, evening primrose, garlic, hawthorn, milk thistle, saw palmetto and turmeric. I wouldn't hesitate to eat bilberries, blueberries, or cranberries every morning with my bran flakes, although, I confess, I do not. I do, though, chomp almost every day on celery like Bugs Bunny chomps on carrots. (What's up, Doc? I'll be glad to tell you!) And I rival Bugs in carrot consumption, too.

Evening primrose is best for adult women as premenstrual tension nears. Some women take a daily maintenance dose; some double or quadruple the dosage as their periods near. Heavy drinkers and men with prostate problems also might want to take it regularly.

Garlic, along with chives, leeks, and onions, can be a daily delight if you have breath mints handy. You can eat hawthorn every day, too, but I'd recommend doing so only if you're an older person with heart problems or a child with attention deficit/hyperactivity disorder. You can also apparently safely indulge in standardized horse chestnut extracts every day (some older books claim the seed is poisonous!), but you may need it only if you're worried about varicose veins. Milk thistle is another everyday item, but only if you're a heavy drinker or are exposed regularly to cigarette smoke, industrial pollution, airport fumes, and other nasty carcinogenic cocktails.

Native Americans certainly regarded saw palmetto as a food, but I've never been able to acquire a taste for its smelly berries. I take it supplementally. Finally, that yellow streak you see on my back is not because I'm afraid of consuming turmeric every day; it's because I often *do* take turmeric, though rarely on a daily basis. Mainly, I use it as a spice and as a standardized supplement.

The more medicinal plants are echinacea, ginkgo biloba, horse chestnut, kava kava, and St. John's wort. Echinacea is definitely a treatment for colds and infections, but herbal authorities disagree over whether it works preventively. I think it does, which is why I take it often during the flu season. Whether it can protect you all year long is open to debate. Some evidence suggests our immune systems might get used to it if taken for a lengthy period. While I take it preventively during flu season, I don't do so for a long time and am not yet ready to endorse regular, daily consumption. Ginkgo's best for people in their forties and older, especially if they're genetically targeted for its best applications.

Kava is essentially a food or a food/beverage, but I don't think my ancestors ingested it as they did coffee and tea. It has its own specific purpose, but daily use is okay. St. John's wort might be the most medicinal of all the herbs in this book. It's strictly a medicine, not a food. Take it only for the symptoms I indicate and for no longer than six weeks at a time. Then consult with a practitioner schooled in phytomedicines.

Plants in Perspective

Because I'm an herb expert, you might think I advocate herbs above all else. I don't. Herbs and the supplements made from them aren't the be-all and end-all of a healthy lifestyle. They're close to the top, but I don't rank them first. Diet and exercise take precedence, in my view. Stress reduction demands top billing, too.

Diet and nutrient supplementation. Good overall nutrition is of utmost importance. You should be moderate in all that you do except varying your diet. Eat a broad mix of antioxidant-rich fruits and vegetables, nuts, grains, wild greens, and, when feasible, wild game and wild fish. The better my diet meets these specifications, the less I feel a need for herbal supplements.

Exercise. I begin and end every day with a progression of back exercises, and I'm fanatical about getting at least a little physical activity

Lay That Silver Bullet Down
(Sung to the tune of "Lay That Pistol Down")

The only herb I take
On every single day
Cel'ry lowers uric acid
And keeps the gout away.
The drug, it costs a whole lot more
That allopurinol,
Cel'ry stops gout in its tracks
Really works, y'all.
Feel them coming on
Bronchitis, colds and flu
I'll take echinacea
The herb I always choose.
I also take the garlic
Almost every day
The grandkids, they kinda shy away
But it keeps the germs at bay
Bilberries, blueberries, and craisins
And the vine that they call Vitis
That's where we get the raisins
To fight the maculitis.
I often memorize my lines
But sometimes I do not
That's when I take my ginkgo
But...you got it, I forgot!
Travel is bedraggling
Airport's such a mess
That's when I take my kava
To mellow down the stress
Depressed, Zoloft is oft used
But old Saint John is best
Puts you in a better mood
With fewer side effects.

Prostate glands, they grow
As old age comes along
But with my saw palmetto,
I don't tinkle all night long.
Synthetic drugs, they disturb
Your cardiac synergies
But hawthorn is a gentle herb
That stops the heart disease
Celebrex done killed ten men
But not me—what me worry?
When my arthritis starts kickin' in,
I just up my dose of curry
Turmeric's anti-arthritic
And has its saving grace
Like Celebrex it inhibits
That cylcooxygenase
And if you're overlivin'
One herb that you should choose
Milk thistle saves your liver
From the mushrooms and the booze.
Compression socks atrocities!
I prefer horse chestnut pills
Slow down those varicosities
Better than drugs will
Medicine men, they often talk
In tongues and alphabets
EPO for BPH
GLA for PMS
Been taking evening primrose,
Two decades, more or less,
And I suspect most everyone knows,
I ain't got PMS

in between. I try to do two 15-minute sessions on the stationary bike every day. If I'm stressed or something upsets me, I'll do more. Ride away your rage, I say. I also stroll through my woods and dig in the herbal vineyard, the six-acre Green Farmacy Garden I've created with Peggy, my wife, and our kids behind our home in Fulton, Maryland.

Stress reduction. My daily walks through the vineyard enable me to commune with my plants and to pay my respects to nature. Such visits instill an amazing sense of serenity to mind and body. I further cultivate calmness when I do my back exercises. A cup of herbal tea in our garden gazebo or the sunroom is a wonderful relaxer, too. Toward evening, I'll sip an herbal tincture, both relaxing and medicinal.

An overwhelming mountain of well-documented research establishes that good diet, regular exercise, and stress management are the keys to preventing disease, staving off the effects of aging, and maintaining health. The lack of all three are huge contributors to our major killers. Together, the trio probably saves many more lives in this country than the $150 billion worth of pharmaceuticals manufactured every year.

chapter two

Best Herbal Medicine, Best Herbal Bargain

WHEN I TOSS A SALAD or dip a ladle into a big pot of vegetable soup, I want my greens and herbs untouched: unaltered, unprocessed. I'd rather they were fresh from my organic backyard, where they're nurtured, watched like babies, and harvested with my own two hands. When it comes to my tea, I'm a purist about the herbs and mints that go into my daily drink. They must be pristine.

I've grown every plant in this book except one (bilberry, but I'm working on it) and dozens upon dozens more. I've made my own tinctures and have treated my own wounds with homemade herbal poultices and compresses. Even though I regret the cost, compared with impure, chemically grown herbs, fruits, and vegetables, I fervently believe in the superiority of whole, organic, unprocessed food plants.

Given these predilections, you'll be surprised to learn that, with only a few exceptions, I don't believe that whole, unprocessed herbs necessarily represent the best way to derive therapeutic benefit from medicinal plants.

Yup, the ol' caretaker of Father Nature's "Farmacy" takes sup-

(continued on page 28)

Standardized Science, Unstandardized Art

I doubt you'll ever catch me taking a supplement of standardized coffee extract. So far, the herbal medicine caffeine I dispense to myself with coffee comes unstandardized, unpurified, unisolated. The same goes for tea. And the same goes for a cup of cocoa.

Part of the reason is the whole experience. There's nothing like sitting down to a steaming cup of coffee. Or tea. Or cocoa. The warm liquid trickles down your esophagus and fills your belly. The aroma's invisible fingers, so inviting and exciting, slither through the air and wiggle their way into your nose. Even the preparation—warming the water, heating the milk—primes your senses to receive the phytochemical fix.

But that's not all. There's an indefinable something in the drink that does not—cannot—transfer to an isolated, standardized extraction. Somehow, those xanthine alkaloids in coffee, tea, and cocoa work better in a simple home-brewed extraction rather than in a fancy distillation process. I feel the same way about most of my herbal teas and liqueurs, too.

The Measure of Medicine

As much as I want to tell you that phytomedicine is a rigid science with rigid protocols that demand rigidly dependable dosages, I really can't. In my mind, I adamantly believe that people generally should take standardized herbal supplements. My heart, though, still tugs at whole, unadulterated foods. So do my tastebuds. (As an aside, you may not even need herbs if you're sure that your diet, exercise, and stress management programs are satisfactory. But that's not the case with most of us.)

It's tough to explain when you should take the supplements and when you might, instead, rely on whole foods. I have a knowledge of herbs and an intuitive feel that took decades to acquire. Most people just want to know what works, when it works, and, sometimes, why. I wish I could fashion a few hard-and-fast rules, but I can't. The best I can do is offer a few examples.

By and large, when I'm on the road and don't have access to my garden, I prefer standardized supplements. Sure, I'll nibble on garlic, onion, and other herbs if I can, but I rely on standardized supplements. At home, I more often take the "food farmacy" approach, leaning on whole plants and herbs for my daily phytochemical dosages. One big exception is celery seed, which, as you'll soon read in chapter 4, has kept me from getting agonizing attacks of gout for more than three years. (Another is saw palmetto; I hate the taste of the berries.) Because I can't fool with gout, I almost always, except when experimenting, take supplements.

Using yourself as a guinea pig is ill-advised, but it's taught me that chomping on four celery stalks protects me from gout just as well as the supplements—so far. Drinking celery juice does the same thing—again, so far. I've been incredibly lucky. Given all the variables that determine a plant's phytochemical content, though, I can never know for sure when or if food farmacy will work. I can bet the farm, though, that swallowing two standardized supplements will keep my big toe free of pain.

If you have gout, you also need to know the amount of celery's active ingredients to which your body will respond. You might need more than me. Or less. Setting dosages by the stalk doesn't give us much of a point of reference. Is it a big stalk or a little one? Do you have green celery or white celery? With a standardized supplement, we can be much more certain and precise.

Don't deny yourself the pleasure of celery juice, celery soup, and whole celery, and even celery seed on an English muffin. Eat and drink to your heart's content. If you consume enough, perhaps you'll stave off gout attacks. Standardized supplements, though, are a better bet.

Choosing Not to Choose?

With other therapeutic plants, I generally go the food farmacy route at home, too—so long as no immediate medical need arises. Unless a cold comes up, I eat unstandardized whole cloves of garlic almost daily instead of taking garlic supplements. If you cannot (or will not) eat garlic every day, you had better look for a good standardized supplement. I dump curry in my recipes rather than swallow turmeric capsules—again, barring some exigency. If I had fresh bilberries, I'd eat them in lieu of taking them in supplemental form. Sometimes, though, I'll help myself to a double-dose of fresh blueberries, expecting approximately the same phytomedicinal effect that I'd get from half as many bilberries.

Granted, I don't know exactly how much of the various active ingredients I'm getting. With food farmacy, you never do. I suspect, though, that the

(continued)

Standardized Science, Unstandardized Art—Continued

unique chemical mixes in food, those blends of phytocompounds that not even the most careful extraction could preserve, are closer to what my genes expect. To an extent, I suppose you could say I'm also hedging my bets, just in case some active ingredients lost in the standardization process turn out to be important.

I readily acknowledge that this answer is inadequate. Perhaps once the medical industry pays more than lip service to phytochemical research, we'll gain a more complete understanding. Until then, I'm sticking with my self-designed program and getting the best of both worlds—the wholesome, healthful goodness of food farmacy and the therapeutic power of standardized supplements.

plements—lots of them. And they're the same ones that you can find in any good health food store.

Sure, I've got a lot of echinacea growing out in my Green Farmacy Garden. The surrounding forest is well-endowed with introduced goldenseal, too. But when I come down with a cold or infection, I almost never harvest either. You just can't know, without lab analyses, the concentration of immunity-strengthening ingredients they contain. And besides, I hate to sacrifice those gorgeous flowers just to get at their roots.

Similarly, I'm voracious about my vineyard-grown garlic, eating it both fresh and aged, raw, cooked, and juiced. But especially when I'm traveling, I also swallow garlic capsules, whose contents are extracted and processed somewhere far, far from my backyard. To build mental musculature and help fend off Alzheimer's disease, I swear by ginkgo biloba, but I rarely consume the leaves of my own ginkgo trees. That could be dangerous for some people, especially if you're sensitive to poison ivy. Besides, I'd need dozens of leaves for just a couple of doses.

All things considered, standardized, store-bought phytomedicinal supplements tend to be more medicinally effective and more qualitatively reliable than whole herbs, whether homegrown, purchased in bulk, or ground up and stuffed into capsules. Efficient, easy to take, and economical, they're the best bet for anyone who isn't intimately knowledgeable about therapeutic plants.

I have only one qualification to my blanket statement. And it's a big one: You have to know what you're getting. You cannot just go to a store and buy any old phytochemical supplement. The smart use of herbs demands that you acquire some smarts about herbs.

The Standardization of Excellence

Little more than a decade ago, I was an ardent advocate of completely natural, unrefined herbs—just the crude plant, steeped in alcohol or vinegar or crushed up into tablets and capsules. I defended my stance even though I constantly encountered sometimes horrendous, quantitative (and thus qualitative) variations in their phytochemicals, the plant chemicals that give them their medicinal value. From species to species, garden to garden, harvest to harvest, the phytochemical content often fluctuated by anywhere from twofold to tenfold. Sometimes, it varied a hundredfold. Nevertheless, I remained a proponent of unrefined crude herbs.

Then one day I read about a subspecies of thyme and the amount of a certain chemical it supposedly contained. Each and every sample was grown within the same square meter of land. One individual plant in that square meter had an impressive 13,900 ppm (parts per million) of the chemical. Another held virtually zero. The other samples measured everything in between. Same soil, same climate, same subspecies. And that was for just one of the thousands of chemicals, many of them medicinal, in this herb.

Thyme, if you will, ran out on my tolerance of phytochemical fluctuations. I started to comprehend how standardization could improve the reliability of herbal medicines.

It's not hard to understand why such great discrepancies occur. You and I belong to the same species, yet we naturally exhibit tremendous differences in our body chemistries. So it is with herbs.

The phytochemical quality of a plant hinges on many variables:

the species, the weather, the soil, the care and tending given, the time of harvest, and the intervening presence of insects, deer, groundhogs, and any other herbivore that might munch on your garden. These factors and others lay the groundwork while the plant is alive. After the harvest, you've got to consider length of storage before processing; exposure to air, contamination, heat, moisture, and sunlight; method of processing; and who knows what else.

To accurately assess a plant's medicinal potential, I became convinced, we needed some way to assure a consistent potency to every batch. Phytochemicals aren't magic. Their mere presence doesn't guarantee success. Usually, a little dab won't do it. A certain amount is required to induce a certain change, and anything less just won't work. (In a few rare cases, a little dab will at least help. If, for example, you're deficient in some vitamins, it seems that every little bit counts.)

Imagine the uncertainty and insanity that would ensue if we couldn't count on the medicinal content of each pill in a bottle of prescription tablets. Or if people with diabetes had to cross their fingers and guess the amount of insulin that filled a syringe. What if they couldn't be certain that the insulin they purchased yesterday was as potent as the vial they bought last month? Without our knowing what to expect, nonstandardized herbs would be less likely to claim their rightful place as superior, safer substitutes for a good many man-made pharmaceuticals.

Pulling Out the Potency

The process of standardization resolves the dilemma. With proper standardization, unlike with the raw, pulverized plant or a simple extract, you know two things:

1. You're getting a certain quantity of the plant.
2. You're getting a certain quantity of one or more of the plant's phytochemicals.

A simple extract is just an herb in concentrated form, and anybody can make one. You do it every time you brew a cup of coffee, for example. You use hot water as a solvent to draw certain compounds out of the ground-up coffee beans. You also expect a certain physiological benefit: You want to wake your tired carcass up and get the day going.

Not too many of us want to relinquish our morning coffee in favor of a few caffeine capsules. That's just one of numerous instances in which the whole, unstandardized crude herb is preferable to its standardized equivalent. When seeking a medicinal or therapeutic effect, though, the average person generally needs an assurance that only a standardized supplement can provide.

Standardizing an herb can provide so-called guaranteed-potency extractions—consistent, measurable levels of one or more active ingredients. Herbal insiders can bicker among themselves over which chemical or which method is best, but the outcome basically remains the same: In every dose, you get a specific amount or amounts of one or more of the plant's many medicinal constituents.

There's a practical aspect to consider, too. In many cases, you have to consume impossibly large quantities of a natural, unrefined herb to get the equivalent beneficial effect of a standardized supplement. Let's say you're interested in saw palmetto for your prostate. In standardized form, you'd take a couple of capsules daily that contain a known level of phytosterols and/or fatty acids. With a supplement made just from crushed-up saw palmetto berries, you might conceivably have to choke down two dozen or so tablets every day. Or you might have to knock back an ounce or more of an alcohol-based saw palmetto tincture. As you can see on the labels, tincture dosages are usually measured with an eye dropper. And even if you could afford a shot's worth of tincture every day, you still might not be getting most of the desired phytochemicals.

The Principal Principle

My first rule for buying medicinal herbs wisely, then, is to stick with standardized brands. Many, but by no means all, plant experts have come to agree on the need to standardize our herbal "farmacy." Some clinical herbalists and naturopaths remain opposed, though, and they state their case quite passionately. I should address two of their arguments:

Cost. Critics claim that standardized extracts cost more. On a purely superficial level, they're right. The whole herb, pulverized and encapsulated, will almost always be cheaper than the standardized version. But, whether with a trowel or a calculator, I always like to dig a little deeper.

If price were the only argument, I'd still conclude that the trade-off is worthwhile, for when we assess cost based on effective dosage of the major active ingredients, the standardized extract clearly is the better bargain. Compared against an unstandardized extract, a tincture, and the whole crude, crushed herb, you get a bigger medicinal bang for the buck.

A standardized ginkgo extract, for example, costs less than $20 a month, as Michael T. Murray, N.D., a naturopathic doctor and one of natural medicine's foremost researchers, noted back in 1996, but the same amount of active ingredient from an alcohol-free commercial tincture costs nearly $500 monthly. St. John's wort, standardized at 0.3 percent hypericin, is less than $20 a month; the alcohol tincture, in contrast, is more than $700. Standardized saw palmetto also costs less than $20 a month, while the alcohol tincture runs you one big Ben Franklin.

Phytochemical synergy. An even more fundamental concern is the integrity and effectiveness of the herbal medicine. Lately, critics have charged that extracting and standardizing isolates certain phytochemicals and robs us of others that are possibly therapeutic.

Theoretically, I suppose, that's true. If we increase one phytochemical, another one must be reduced to compensate. By and large, though, if we are standardizing an herb properly and not just spiking, we don't isolate one compound and filter out everything else. The process reduces the entire plant to a concentrated form, based on measurements of one or more key elements. Generally, when we concentrate one biologically active substance, we usually concentrate closely related chemicals, too, in proportion with the target phytochemicals. We end up with more of the intended chemical and more of its companion constituents. Usually, that means more of the synergistic, therapeutic ingredients that nature intended.

What's wrong with aiming for that main magical, medicinal ingredient? Plenty. If the worst thing about whole herbs is their wide, ever-fluctuating phytochemical content, the best thing is the very existence of so many diverse, biologically active compounds. I'm the first to argue that it is often wrong to single out one chemical as the be-all, end-all ingredient. Dozens of other closely related active compounds usually are present in a plant, and I prefer that they remain present in any supplement. To produce the therapeutic benefit for which the plant is known, in many cases, they work with one another synergistically or additively. Singling out one of them may very well rob us of the plant's full medicinal potential. Our bodies (our genes, that is) know these substances not as isolated chemicals but as they appear in nature.

Here's an extreme analogy: How healthy would we be if science had isolated thiamin (vitamin B_1) and disregarded all other B-complex vitamins? Even the worst nutritionist advises taking a mixture of the whole complex so as not to upset natural ratios. If we just took thiamin, we'd lack vitamin B_2, vitamin B_3, vitamin B_6, and vitamin B_{12}, not to mention folic acid and other nutritional partners. We'd be goners.

I wonder if we've made just such a mistake by focusing on beta-carotene, just one of a whole class of plant pigments that have antioxidant and nutritional qualities, at the expense of all the other carotenoids. Carotenoids are composed of a whole class of yellow to deep red pigments that are found in plants of which beta-carotene is only one member.

And could we have done the same with vitamin E? In nature, a whole group of chemicals called tocopherols and tocotrienols make up a sort of vitamin E complex. But the supplement we commonly buy, DL-tocopherol acetate, is actually a synthetic imitation of a single tocopherol. Are we making the right choice for our health by taking this single substance?

But what if there is no correct choice? I'd like to posit the radical theory that both sides are right and wrong simultaneously. We need *all* of the tocopherols, all of the tocotrienols, all of the carotenoids, and all of the B-complex vitamins. I'll bet that a natural vitamins mix of related compounds is better (and better for us) than an incomplete isolate. One day, in a future where a vitamin E-complex is common-

(continued on page 38)

Farmaceutical Forms

You can enjoy the medicinal benefits of whole herbs, whether cultivated under your own careful watch or bought in bulk from a store, in several ways—from meals and drinks to tinctures, poultices, and compresses.

Meals

My favorite way, of course, is in food, whether as a spice, garnish, condiment, or main ingredient. Here and there throughout these pages, you'll see what I loosely refer to as recipes. I cook, but I'm not a great one by any definition. Unless I'm following a recipe strictly, only rarely do I use a measuring spoon or a measuring cup for its intended purpose. A pinch of this, a dash or two of that, a big handful of something else—guesswork guides me. No recipe is ever quite the same. Usually, the meal is very good. Every once in a while, it's not. Either way, it always surprises me.

Teas

Beginning as soon as I can with spring's new growth, throughout the summer, and right until fall's last harvest, I make tea with fresh, right-from-the-plant herbs. As a matter of fact, here in Maryland I can find basal rosettes of some flavorful mints all year long.

You can certainly use dried herbs, but a lot of the aromatic compounds are lost in the drying process. (You can even crack open capsules of powdered herbs.) The brew from fresh plants usually tastes better, though, and the whole process is much more enjoyable. Just keep in mind that fresh herbs are about 80 percent water and 20 percent phytochemicals. Reverse the numbers for the approximate composition of dried herbs.

Because tea recipes typically call for the dry form, you need a general conversion rule: To get roughly the same potency, use about four times as much fresh herb as you would dry herb. To make a tea that's as therapeutic as it is thirst-quenching, you'll probably require a refresher course in how to brew. Most people simply pour hot water over a tea bag, squeeze the bag with a teaspoon a few times, and drink up. Medicinal tea isn't made so instantly. You have a choice of two methods. If leaves and flowers comprise the tea material, use the infusion method. If you're working with roots and stems, make a decoction.

Infusion. Pour boiling water in a cup and let the herbs steep until the water cools. Allow the water to draw out the phytochemicals for some 10 to 20 minutes.

Decoction. Roots, stems, and bark release their medicinal compounds more reluctantly. Put the desired amount of plant in water and boil it on the stove for 10 to 20 minutes.

And then there's the sun method—steeping aromatic plants in a jar of water on a hot, bright day. I've enjoyed sun teas occasionally, but they always bring to mind the hay infusions we made to prepare for labs in the old days. To culture amoebae and other microscopic amazements, we'd steep hay in water and let it sit in the sun. If I could examine my old sun teas under a microscope, I think I'd find a host of interesting protozoans swimming around in there.

Tinctures

The name may conjure up thoughts of alchemy and witches' potions, but medicinal martini might be a little more apt. The classic before-dinner drink is essentially a hydroalcoholic tincture of onion (or olive, depending on your preferences, although both are good food farmaceuticals).

A tincture is just another liquid-based way of extracting some therapeutic potential from a plant. Instead of steeping the herb for 10 to 20 minutes, as you would a tea, you wait for a week. And in place of boiling water, you substitute your favorite alcohol. I'm rather fond of vodka, but pure ethanol will do, too.

If you're not comfortable with alcohol, use vinegar. It draws out some phytochemicals just as well. You can use an alcohol-based tincture to complement and strengthen herbal teas and juices. A vinegar-based culinary tincture is great as a salad dressing or as an extra ingredient in soups, stews, and other recipes.

Amounts to use vary widely, anywhere from several drops to a dropperful or more. With homemade tinctures, you're generally on your own for how much to take. Commercially made tinctures often suggest a dosage on their labels.

Unless consumed in great quantity, a tincture doesn't typically give you a

(continued)

big shot of phytochemical medicine. However, the active plant ingredients do enter your bloodstream a bit faster, and a lot of people find it easier to swallow a liquid rather than a couple of capsules.

Tinctures are best for herbs whose therapeutic activities depend largely on their aromatic constituents. These volatile compounds are readily lost in bulk, ground, and powdered forms unless processed and packaged carefully with antioxidants. Tinctures capture and preserve them a little better. Among my baker's dozen of recommended herbs, those whose health-influencing properties stem at least in part from their aromatic compounds are celery seed, turmeric, and garlic. St. John's wort works well as a tincture, too. Have you ever seen a martini with a garlic clove before? I haven't, but I think I'll experiment with one tonight. That's part of the beauty of this form of herbal medicine. Do-it-yourselfers can enjoy tinkering with their own tinctures. Pick an herb and see what happens.

Whether you use alcohol or vinegar, the instructions are the same. Measure 2 ounces of dried herb (or 1 handful of fresh herb) for every pint of liquid, and just let the mixture sit. I prefer to cover it and keep it in a dark, cool spot. Every once in a while, stop by and stir it a little. After about a week, strain the liquid (discard the sediment) and store it in a bottle.

Poultices and Compresses

Sometimes, the best way in is from without. Compresses and poultices are two time-honored topical methods to apply a phytochemical, usually to an injury or another problem site. In most cases, you want to fight an infection or speed healing, but I'm sure the body puts to good use elsewhere all the healing compounds it absorbs.

Belatedly, science is discovering that many substances are absorbed transdermally, meaning through the skin. We'll probably learn of more. Right now, though, there's more scientific evidence supporting internal use of Duke's Dozen than their topical application. The best evidence leads me to conclude that none of Duke's Dozen can be used to full effect strictly as a poultice or compress. That's not to say they may not have some value. You should definitely experiment. In folk medicine, some of my 13 herbs have indeed been used topically.

Mashed garlic and mashed turmeric, for example, have been applied as poultices to help wounds heal. I have even used garlic poultices on infections, with good results. Similarly, mashed horse chestnut has been placed directly on a bruise or a site of swelling. A poultice of celery or turmeric might help tame inflammation. I've never tested either, but their use makes sense. Compresses of St. John's wort oil or alcoholic tincture have been placed on burns and arthritic joints. (If you try celery or St. John's wort in this manner, stay out of the sun. They might cause photodermatitis.)

Echinacea, my number two herb after celery seed extract, boasts a whole array of often overlooked topical uses. Europeans consider it handy for burns, ulcers, varicosities, wounds, and such skin conditions as inflammatory lesions from allergic dermatitis, herpes simplex, and psoriasis. Historically, the plant has also been used for carbuncles, cellulitis, chicken pox, decubitis (pressure ulcer), erysipelas (a bacterial infection characterized by fever and inflammation and redness of the skin and subcutaneous tissues), folliculitis (inflammation of a follicle, ordinarily in reference to a hair follicle), furuncles (also known as boils), gangrene, paronychia (inflammation involving the folds of tissue surrounding the nail), scarlet fever, smallpox, and stings. Newer lab studies suggest that phytochemicals in echinacea might protect skin against ultraviolet damage from a sunburn. I've never tried any of these applications personally, but the research looks good.

How might you take advantage of an herb's therapeutic touch? Creams, lotions, and ointments are difficult to make at home, but compresses and poultices are easy enough. For a compress, dip a clean cloth in the herbal liquid of choice; tea or tincture, infusion, decoction, alcohol, vinegar—it doesn't matter. Apply the cloth directly to the skin, and change it several times a day.

You can use the compress cloth to hold a poultice in place. To make a poultice, just grab a handful of fresh, chopped plant material (if it's dry, wet it). To coax out the medicinal compounds, boil, steam, chew, or hammer on the plant, then mold it into a small ball and put it right on the skin. To make the poultice easier to handle, you might want to make an herbal dough of sorts, using one part of the softened herb with three parts of either water, alcohol, or vinegar. Thicken it with as much flour as necessary.

place, we may look back with a sad smile on the days of man-made DL-tocopherol acetate.

Herbal equivalents abound. It makes no sense, to give one example, to isolate a single sulfur compound in garlic. The result would be less effective than a standardized whole extract—and more expensive, to boot. Yet the supplement industry really is expending energy on this very endeavor. Don't buy it, literally or figuratively. Nutrient profiteers are doing the same with St. John's wort: Some American experts are pushing hypericin as the main active ingredient, while their German counterparts tout a compound called hyperforin. Each has some science on its side.

And each seems to lack some holistic common sense. Once more, I'd like to propose a simplistic notion: It's not just one or another active ingredient—or even something else that has not yet been identified. It's *all* of them, each with its own peculiar contribution to the plant's therapeutic value. Keep this in mind if you ever hear of a successful attempt to isolate just one of the various complex carbohydrates in echinacea, just one of the essential oil terpenoids or phthalides in celery, just one of the flavonoids in hawthorn, or just one of the phytosterols or fatty acids in saw palmetto.

Tincture Talk

Some herbal authorities maintain that tinctures retain more of a plant's full range of biochemicals. In certain cases, this is true. But usually not. For most herbs, a dry standardized extract contains higher concentrations of the primary ingredients. Complex chemical analyses, according to Dr. Murray, all show that standardized extracts, compared with tinctures, typically contain both higher amounts and a wider range of phytochemicals.

The frequent exception would be those pleasing herbs whose therapeutic effects rely on their aromatic or alcohol-soluble ingredients, especially volatile chemicals that are easily lost. Usually, tinctures retain these delicate compounds better than other forms. This is why, for instance, I frequently take both the tincture and tablet form of echinacea when the flu is going around. The tincture contains more of certain active ingredients, the standardized supplement more of certain others.

Overall, though, for most herbs, a dry standardized extract provides higher concentrations, because a liquid generally cannot hold the same amount of active ingredients. And if the manufacturing process is done well, encapsulating an herb will better preserve those active ingredients. Dr. Murray points to complex chemical analyses showing that standardized extracts, compared with tinctures, contain both higher amounts and a wider range of plant chemicals.

Into the Herb Store: Let the Buyer Be Wary

Even if you accept the superiority of standardized supplements, you're not yet fully herbally empowered. Your initial trips into an herb store still will be absolutely bewildering—if not frightening. There are hundreds of different products offered by dozens of different companies. How do you know what to get?

Education is your best ally. Never cease to ask questions until you're satisfied you can make a thoughtful decision. Question what you read on labels, question store clerks, question different stores, question different manufacturers. When you buy a refrigerator or some other big-ticket item, I doubt that you visit only one store. You go to several. You compare brands, prices, and features. A fridge is a big investment. You want performance, value, and dependability. In purchasing supplements, you're also making a big investment. Good herbs are therapeutic and preventive investments in good health.

So walk into that health food store as if you're entering a car dealership. Better yet, because you'll put these products into your body and expect consistent positive results, stroll on in with the same attitude you'd take to a doctor's office—in need of help and inquisitive, yet skeptical. When you get right down to it, herbal supplements *are* medications.

I can't ensure that you'll buy what's best the first time and every time. All I can do is point out some pitfalls you might encounter on your way and try not to steer you in the wrong direction.

Lessons on the Label

By far your most significant indication of quality is the label. Intentionally or not, it can be quite informative. You just have to decipher what's on it—and what has been left off. Let me illustrate by recounting a phone conversation I had not too long ago.

The caller wanted to know about saw palmetto for prostate enlargement. He was taking the powdered whole fruit and preferred to stick with this supplemental form. Was it as good as what I use, he asked, and how much of it should he take? When I suggested he follow the label's instructions, he countered that no such dosage recommendation—or much of anything else, for that matter—appeared. I told him he should seek another brand.

This information, or lack thereof, immediately told me several things about this particular product. Ideally, a good supplement label should answer each of the following questions. In reality, though, few actually will address all of my criteria directly, so I'll give you a quick lesson in reading between the lines. One way or another, you'll learn how to get a sense of a product's quality.

How much should I take and how often? Since 1994, when the U.S. Food and Drug Administration (FDA) relaxed its choke hold, supplement suppliers have been allowed to recommend daily dosages. Don't accept any assertion otherwise. The caller's product was thus either outdated, or its manufacturer was still too chicken to suggest an amount.

If a company doesn't wish to make recommendations about its own brand, would it not be litigiously foolish of me to make one on its behalf? More important, you, the consumer, are left in the dark with absolutely no idea of how much to take—or how much you're putting inside your body.

What exactly is in this, and is it standardized? As I told my caller, even though I have a saw palmetto plant in my greenhouse and pounds of its stinking (literally!) fruit in my book room, I prefer standardized supplements to the whole berry. I then briefly explained why: I want to know what I'm ingesting and how much.

A good label gives you that information very plainly. It's supposed to make you nod your head, not scratch it.

His berry powder, according to the label, contained 90 percent fatty acids and sterols. Hmmm, I thought. What sterols? Which fatty acids? What is the amount of each? And what's in that remaining 10 percent? Though his label, in this regard, read like most of those on bottles of standardized saw palmetto, you still need specifics. Granted, a supplier can't list all the thousands of compounds in a plant. But the more information the manufacturer provides, the more useful the supplement becomes.

A quick glance at the fine print should also tell you whether you're getting the whole plant, part of the plant (which part?), or an extract. If the latter, is the extract standardized? Standardized for what? It should cite the major active ingredient or ingredients.

Don't fall for phonies. Right up front, you should learn the plant's scientific name. If only a common name appears and you've never heard of it, don't buy the product. If only some bogus botanical designation appears and you're not familiar with it, don't buy the product. Some unscrupulous dealers intentionally use obscure or contrived names.

Refuse a ratio. Expect to see how much of the active ingredients each capsule contains. Look for a percentage; don't settle for a ratio. If you read that a St. John's wort supplement contains a 10 to 1 ratio of hyperforin to hypericin, all you'd know is that there's a lot more of one compound than another. You still don't know if the supplement is high or low in either.

What else is in it and why? Did the manufacturer add antioxidants or other preservatives? Pulverized whole herbs, in particular, are very perishable without antioxidant protection. The label should also tell you about added fillers or the inclusion of any other herb or herbs, especially from an unlike species.

Multiple-herb formulas are a hot trend in the supplement business these days. The ill-informed thinking must be, If one is good, minuscule amounts of two dozen others must be better. Laugh at the lunacy in this logic, and buck the trend. Unless you've learned of some strong scientific rationale for the blend, beware. If a supplement contains two or three or more herbs, you need to know why.

Here's why you should know: Within a species or group of

(continued on page 44)

Growing Pains and Pleasures

Most people don't have the luxury of growing fresh herbs and ingesting them straight from the garden. I do, and I indulge myself whenever I have the time. Gardening is an almost spiritual endeavor—a way to feel as one with the Earth, a rewarding hobby, a good form of exercise, and an economical way to delight your tastebuds and nourish yourself with nutrients at their freshest.

If I can grow the herbs in this book, so can you. And even though you usually should stick with standardized supplements for the best medicinal effect, I urge you to try your hand at cultivating these plants. Sow them, grow them, know them. They can be good friends.

You don't need six acres for your own herbal haven. A sunny back porch or windowsill will do. Not all of Duke's Dozen will thrive in a pot on your kitchen window, but some will survive. Echinacea, for instance, is a beautiful ornamental that's easy to raise. Ginkgo biloba is so hardy that many refer to it as a living fossil, and I've even seen beautiful, potted bonsai Ginkgo. (I don't recommend home preparations of ginkgo, however, especially if you're sensitive to poison ivy.) Garlic and its relatives—onions, leeks, and chives—can sprout inside the house, but grow them outdoors if you want their pungent roots.

Saw palmetto, a tropical, could be grown indoors like an ornamental palm, but it requires a very warm windowsill or, ideally, a greenhouse. The same is true of turmeric, a member, like cardamom, of ginger's *Zingiberaceae* family. Some trees, like ginkgo, hawthorn, and horse chestnut, might be grown as bonsai plants. If the sill is dry and very sunny, try nursing to life some St. John's wort. I've never been able to get seeded potted plants of St. John's wort to flower on a windowsill, but I'll bet the better gardeners out there can. Whether the weed blossoms or not, though, be sure to show visitors its purplish pores, known descriptively as the blood of St. John.

Therapeutic herbs not in my top 13 that should do well indoors include aloe vera, the burn plant, and oregano, a potent antioxidant. To get started, you might try some parsley; while you're at it, complete the quartet with some sage, rosemary, and thyme. Other good indoor growers include dill, well-known as a remedy for gas; rosemary, chock-full of antioxidant nutrients and a potential ally in staving off Alzheimer's disease; basil, another breath freshener as well as a headache remedy and insect repellent; peppermint, one of our best sources for cool, stomach-calming menthol; and fennel, another natural indigestion aid.

If you have some ground to till and tend, by all means grow garlic, onions, leeks, and chives. Other herbs outside of Duke's Dozen that should grow well include goldenseal—a natural antibiotic, good for colds and infections—which grows best in the shade; lemon balm, a virus-fighter that doubles as a mild sedative; oregano, a superb spice loaded with antioxidants; and valerian, one of the most powerful herbal stress busters we have.

Healthy Harvest

Gardening goes far beyond the scope of this book, I'm afraid. But let's say you've planted a "green farmacy" of your own and now have a harvest of feisty, full-bloom plants ready to offer their remedial services. What do you do with them?

First off, the fresh leaves of culinary and edible species make delicious additions to recipes. Why reach for those tiny tins in the spice rack when you can clip off a few fresh, fragrant leaves and toss them right in the pot? If you're gathering fresh herbs for food, collect them in plastic bags to help preserve their moisture. If you're harvesting to preserve them in some fashion, use paper bags to decrease the risk of mold growth.

Savor the distinctive aromatic presence of your fresh harvest. Keep in mind, though, that the scent is a sign that the herb is starting to lose some of its volatile compounds. With each sniff, some medicinal molecules abandon the harvested plant and head for your olfactory senses. The escape occurs, unavoidably, as soon as you remove the leaves or bark or other part of the plant from the living plant. You'll lose more, and somewhat change the plant's chemical profile, when you dry the herb, no matter what method you choose. Light, heat, and mere exposure to the air around us all drain an herb of its potency. More strength dissipates when you dry the herb, whether you leave it out in the sun, bake it in an oven, or nuke it in the microwave.

In ascending order of potency preservation, I'd follow sun drying with low-temperature closed-oven drying, microwave drying, shade drying, and freeze-

(continued)

Growing Pains and Pleasures—Continued

drying. Few people, myself included, are equipped to freeze-dry herbs at home.

Sun drying. Sun drying is simply placing harvested plant material in a location where the heat of the sun is allowed to dry them. I'd say this is the least recommended preservative method, an assertion that admittedly comes not from any quantitative chemical analysis or strictly conducted lab testing, just a gut feeling based on a lot of experience.

Conventional oven drying. If you use a conventional oven, set a low temperature (about 140°F or so) and let the herbs dry only until they're crisp, checking them frequently. This should take a few hours, at most, depending on the herb. Avoid high heat, whether in the oven or elsewhere.

Microwaving. Microwaving is fast and convenient, something almost everyone can do. I suspect that this method preserves much of the heavier, nonvolatile therapeutic compounds. Experiment by microwaving herbs for 30-second intervals using the medium setting. Purists, I'm certain, will turn up their eyebrows at me whether I microwave a medicinal plant or nuke a cold cup of coffee. But I do so with little fear of irradiating myself, and I consider it a reasonable drying method, at least for herbs whose medicinal effect does not originate from volatile aromatic compounds.

species, closely related biochemical compounds often interact synergistically with one another—they work, or work better, together. Evolution made it so. But there usually is no evolutionary reason for synergies among unlike phytochemicals from unlike species—especially if they're from different continents.

Sometimes, a good reason exists. In Chinese, Ayurvedic, and Native American medicines, for instance, treatments may contain a dozen different species or more. I have great respect for some of these traditional combinations. Millennia of empirical experience back them up. But for some Johnny-come-lately combinations, the scientific evidence typically is lacking. Certain mixtures have been tested in a wide array of good studies, but the research done on others would not pass the necessary muster.

I'll be bold enough to say that, in general, the more herbal ingre-

I must caution, though, that I haven't had much luck with drying aromatic herbs. Not long ago, I experimented with the microwave method by drying small bunches of lemon balm and mountain mint. A minute didn't dry the herb entirely. Two minutes dried the plants but still left some green coloring. After three minutes, the herbs were dry enough to crush into a powder, but my nose could hardly distinguish the mountain mint from the lemon balm. I'm guessing that microwave drying destroyed vulnerable aromatic phytochemicals.

Warm shade drying. For warm shade drying, spread harvested herbs out on a screen or some newspapers in a dry, shady spot, ideally away from direct sunlight. Expect to wait about a week.

Storing Dried Herbs

However you decide to dry, you'll know your job is done when the herbs, though still green, wither, stiffen, and become brittle. Store the dried herbs in glass jars with tight-fitting lids, plastic bags, or paper bags in a dark, cool spot. Glass jars are best. Try to keep the leaves, stems, and roots relatively whole; don't crumble or crush them.

dients in a formula, the less likelihood that any good scientific study provides a rationale.

What does this stuff do, and could it hurt me? Make no bones about it: Good herbal supplements are medications. To say otherwise is to lie, or to spout off ignorantly. And as with any medication, you need to know about any possible side effects or any reasons why you shouldn't put it into your body.

You also should get a general sense of what the herb purportedly does. Don't fall for crazy claims. If the label hints at relief from dozens of ills, suggests that herbs do not have side effects, claims that all natural substances are harmless, or alleges that numerous controlled, clinical trials prove the product's efficacy even to the FDA's satisfaction—or if anything similarly ridiculous appears on the package—put it back on the shelf.

Is the label dated? A friend of mine once told me about going to a health food store to purchase an herbal laxative for his mother. He picked up something that turned out to be 10 years old. The sales clerk expressed no concern at all about the product's age. The lack of concern belies a lack of intelligence—and a lack of regard for your well-being.

Herbal supplements don't retain their potency forever. Some might keep longer than others, depending on the plant, the inclusion of preservatives, and other factors we have already discussed. Most manufacturers don't stamp expiration dates or even packaging dates on their products. Sometimes a date appears but is cryptically encoded.

It's time manufacturers included expiration dates in bold print. We need to know when that bottle of capsules was made—last week? Last year? Last decade?

Unfortunately, no hard-and-fast rule exists for how old is too old. Sometimes, scent can give you a sense of age. In giving off an aroma, a harvested herb gives off its aromatic molecules—which could very well be the plant's medicinal molecules. If it has no more aromatic molecules to give off, then that sample has little or no therapeutic potential.

If you crack open a garlic capsule, an onion capsule, or a valerian capsule, it should reek. If you buy an herbal laxative that is supposed to be powerfully aromatic but it lacks that strong smell when you open the bottle, the supplement probably has lost some, if not much, of its medicinal power.

Want a general rule? Okay. Duke winks and thinks, "The best stinks, at least with garlic and valerian."

Can I contact you? A responsible supplement maker, in my view, welcomes customer questions, complaints, and comments. Indeed, the company should encourage such feedback with a tollfree telephone number. At the very least, the label should include a mailing address. I prefer a tollfree support line, but lamentably, you won't find one very often.

Brand. I'm reluctant to make outright endorsements. Instead, I'll give you a general rule of thumb and tell you what my colleagues think.

I'll be very up-front and tell you that my post-retirement employer is Nature's Herbs. It's a good company, in my estimation, with a good reputation and good products. Many other suppliers also offer quality herbs. During my years at the U.S. Department of Agriculture, we had to name at least three dealers we considered reputable. I'll carry that dictum over into my retirement and name a few of the better brands: Bioforce, Eclectic, Enzymatic Therapy, Nature's Herbs, Nature's Way, Phytopharmica, Quanterra, Schwabe, Solaray, and Solgar.

This list, keep in mind, is not comprehensive. I am not suggesting that other brands do not offer quality supplements. Many do. Nor am I making specific endorsements. I'm simply telling you that, according to an informal, thoroughly unscientific survey of some of my most highly regarded colleagues, these companies have earned a reputation for supplying reliable products.

Price. Generally, when dealing with nationally recognized labels, you get what you pay for. Top-notch phytochemical supplements, whether distributed by one of the companies I just cited or another firm, usually do cost more than lesser-quality brands.

Based on everything I've dealt with over the last couple of decades, cut-rate generic and store-brand labels often do not contain enough of the active ingredients to make them real bargains. Properly identifying, growing, harvesting, processing, packaging, and labeling a high-quality herb takes money. If one brand costs substantially less than others, quality often, though not invariably, has been compromised.

In evaluating price, you must do more than compare costs. Again, look at the label. How many pills are in the bottle? How many do you need for the suggested dosage? Is the dosage the same from brand to brand? With less expensive brands, sometimes you must take two or three pills to equal the potency of one pill from a different maker.

Stores and clerks. Input from store clerks can sometimes be helpful. Sometimes, it can be dangerous. In an ideal world, sales people would be intimately familiar with the products they hawk, but we know this isn't always the case. With luck, perhaps you'll chance upon a shop whose employees know their stuff.

So by all means, ask questions. Find out if and why store clerks take the herbs you're interested in. Which brands do they favor? Why? Take all replies, though, with that proverbial grain of salt, if not the whole shaker. Beware of clerks who have a flippant answer for every question, and always ask them the basis for their reply. If a salesperson can't answer a question, can he or she call the manufacturer to get an answer? Can you? Don't be satisfied with one visit to one store. Go to several herb shops.

Taking Herbal Medicines Safely

One reason herbal medicines are comparable to prescription drugs is their well-deserved reputation for safety, earned by being self-tested on people for thousands of years. Besides working as well, or almost as well, as drugs, they're generally better tolerated and freer of adverse reactions. Unwanted side effects from herbs, when they occur, usually aren't as severe, either.

Pharmaceutical antidepressants can cause insomnia, intestinal upset, and weight gain, among other consequences. They may also ruin your sex life. In contrast, the worst that may be said about St. John's wort, nature's antidepressant, is that excessive doses might sensitize your skin to the sun.

Don't conclude, though, that herbal medicine is without risk. It is not. All medications, nature-made or man-made, carry a chance of adverse side effects. Well-known herbs are generally quite safe; highly concentrated extracts are more liable to have minor side effects. Isolated phytochemicals may be a bit more hazardous, but on average they are less likely to cause harm than the synthetics your genes don't know.

Beware Herbal Hysteria

Some herbal adversaries take the above acknowledgment and run with it. Over the course of 1998, the increasing use of phytomedicines was met with a crescendo of warnings, perhaps well-intentioned but definitely not well-informed, about obscure or even nonexistent potential hazards. For example, one widely acclaimed clinical guide faults people for mixing drugs and herbs that may not go well together. Warning about echinacea's extremely remote risk of liver toxicity, it concludes that you shouldn't take it at all if you're on any potentially hepatoxic medications, such as amiodarone, prescribed for irregular heart rhythm; methotrexate, an immune suppressant used in treating rheumatoid arthritis and severe psoriasis, among other conditions; ketoconazole, an antifungal treatment; or if you have an autoimmune disorder like lupus or multiple sclerosis.

I know of no studies showing that echinacea can damage the liver. And I'll wager that more than half the drugs in the *Physicians Desk Reference* pose potential liver problems, at least as indicated by elevated hepatic levels. My question to echinacea's enemies, then, is: What's your point?

The plant's danger in autoimmune disease is hypothetical; no research verifies the possibility. However, many phytochemical experts, myself included, caution against the use of immune-reinforcing herbs if you have an autoimmune disease. By definition, an autoimmune disease is one in which the immune system goes into overdrive against the very body it's designed to protect. It only makes sense that you shouldn't fertilize an already-overactive immune system.

Such negative claims about phytochemical therapy are almost invariably anecdotal, speculative, theoretical, or hyperbolic. The alarmists don't realize it, but their dire warning says more in favor of herbal medicine than against it: They implicitly acknowledge that herbs actually do work. They want proponents to cite supporting clinical trials before we advocate supplementation. I'd like to suggest that the critics sponsor unbiased studies to prove or disprove their unsubstantiated speculations.

In waving red flags, the foes of phytomedicine imply that herbal advocates ignore potential problems and endanger the public. Well, the responsible ones among us certainly do not. My advocacy of herbal medicine is unabashed. Against the average pharmaceutical, I'll bet my bottom dollar on the safety of all 13 herbs in this book—almost half of them are mere foods. And all 13 have proof backing them up.

Practical Advice for Safety and Success

At the same time, though, I don't recommend supplementation lightly, and I'm not going to recommend something known to be risky. I'm duty-bound and honor-bound to report the bad with the good. When you read about the hazardous potential of an herb in this book, you can rest assured that the possibility is real, although probably remote.

As with any medication, you have a big role to play in minimizing any potential peril. Phytochemical supplements are medications, so treat them as such. You can take several measures to help ensure that your herbal adventure is satisfying, successful, and safe.

Don't go it alone. You'll probably be able to pinpoint what herbs are best for a certain condition, but you shouldn't try to identify the problem by yourself. Let a physician do that, then discuss with him or her your desire to treat it with medicinal herbs. Better yet, find a doctor or practitioner who's well-schooled in all the alternative healing arts—not just herbalism but nutrition, naturopathy, exercise, and so on. A multiple-level approach might be best.

Aim high, but start low. Sometimes, a larger dose packs a more powerful punch, but not always. Never assume that if a certain amount is therapeutic, a bigger amount must be even more therapeutic. Taking a huge dose of a phytochemical often has the exact opposite effect than the one you intended. A small dose, for example, might lower blood pressure, but an exceedingly large dose might raise blood pressure, or vice versa.

Don't figure that if one capsule is good, 10 are better. Begin with the lowest possible dosage, perhaps even less than what's suggested, and work up to the full amount. You might need more than is recommended in this book or on a label, but never assume that need.

When I first tested celery seed extract as a gout preventive, I took four capsules a day. That's a lot, and it reflects how much I feared a gout attack. Eventually, though, I realized I had neglected another basic rule of herbal medicine: Take the smallest effective amount. So I adjusted dosages and found that two capsules conferred the same protection as four. Why waste two capsules every day? That translates into twice as many doses to keep me from writhing on the floor with an anguishing pain in my big toe.

Do as directed. Sometimes you'll be advised to take a phyto-chemical product between meals or on an empty stomach. Heed the suggestion. In particular, take it long before or long after you've con-sumed any coffee, tea, or chocolate. Each tends to bind up some herbal ingredients. (The same is true for some synthetic medications.)

Caution: Grapefruit. At least at first, don't wash down herbs, other supplements, or even medications with grapefruit juice. Grape-fruit enhances your body's absorption and utilization of other sub-stances. One study demonstrated that it synergistically increased the effectiveness twofold to sixfold of one out of every three pharmaceu-ticals tested. I'd expect similar results with herbal medications.

Stay on watch. The first time I took a niacin supplement, I thought I was going to die. My face suddenly felt very hot, my heart raced, and I was overcome with a strange tingling sensation. Little welts appeared on my skin. Scared and all alone in my office one Sat-urday morning, I reached for a pen and some paper to write a note about my impending demise to whomever discovered the body. Looking at the label of the vitamin bottle so I could identify my cause of death, I saw the warning about the so-called niacin flush.

Most impressive, I thought. These days, I frequently carry a bottle of niacin with me just to demonstrate the power of natural sup-plements. Whenever I take this form of the B vitamin, I get the flush, often in just a minute or two.

My point, of course, is that these things bring about real physio-logical changes in the body. Whether herbal, nutritional, or pharma-ceutical, you cannot take them casually. Phytochemical supplements sport an outstanding safety record, but you can never really know, at first, how your body will react. You might be allergic to the plant. You might become dizzy, sick to your stomach, or even short of breath.

Just to be on the safe side, no matter what the symptom, your best bet is to call a doctor or allergist. Difficulty breathing is a rare reaction, but if it occurs within 30 minutes or so of taking a new substance—be it natural or pharmaceutical—call 911. You might be experiencing a very rarely seen anaphylactic reaction, the most se-vere form of allergic response. Or you might not be experiencing anything notable at all. In retrospect, it could even be, as was my ini-

Herbally Educated

By reading these words right now, you're taking one of the most important steps you can toward the wise, effective use of phytochemical medicine. Information is everywhere these days, some of it well-reasoned, some of it misleading or outright inaccurate. The more you learn, the more you'll be able to discern the truth, or at least the best-educated consensus of what the truth is, regarding a given herb.

Most of the major health magazines address herbal aspects of health on a continuing basis. They target their articles to the average reader and usually serve as a good source of reasonable information. Popular books about herbs have also proliferated with rising interest in the subject. I'll vouch for the accuracy of my previous book, *The Green Pharmacy*, and can attest to the reliability of *Herbs of Choice* and *Tyler's Honest Herbal*, both by Varro E. Tyler, Ph.D., Sc.D., and *Herbal Medicine*, by R. F. Weiss. Another source is the *1998 Complete German Commission E Monographs*, well-edited by Mark Blumenthal, executive director of the American Botanical Council. Commission E (a German panel of experts roughly equivalent to the U.S. Food and Drug Administration) approaches medicinal plants very conservatively.

The Internet also teems with an abundance of easily accessible information. Again, some of it you can count on; some of it you cannot. Besides my Father Nature's Farmacy, or FNF (also known as Dr. Duke's Photochemical and Ethnobotanical Databases), at www.ars-grin.gov/duke and my Medical Botany Syllabus at www.ars-grin.gov/duke/syllabus, I also am a contributor to the Herb-A-Day column at www.allherb.com. Among other good Web sites are the Alternative Medicine HomePage at www.pitt.edu/~cbw/altm.html; the American Botanical Council at www.herbalgram.org; Ask Dr. Weil at www.hotwired.com/drweil; Natural Health Village at www.naturalhealthvillage.com; and HealthWorld Online at www.healthy.net. Remember, however, that even though the places I've just listed are run by reputable organizations with good track records, Web sites still tend to come and go, and their addresses and sponsors may change from time to time.

tial encounter with niacin, almost amusing. But you never know.

Mix and match carefully. Just because two products are natural doesn't mean they go well together. Compounds in some herbs don't mix well with compounds in other herbs—or even with certain foods. They also may interact unfavorably with medications you might be taking. The two could cancel out or magnify each other's effectiveness. Before you take a new phytochemical product, make sure you're aware of interactions.

Get wired. So far, my herbal desk reference, or HDR, as I call it, is available on the Internet as an important part of my medical botany syllabus. For some 200 herbs, I've gathered together all major legitimately recognized activities, indications, contraindications, and side effects. I revise the HDR constantly, including every report I deem credible, whether good or bad. You'll find it in my Medical Botany Syllabus on the Web at www.ars-grin.gov/duke/syllabus. (For a listing of other recommended Web sites, see "Herbally Educated.")

There's an Art to the Science

If you approach product selection carefully and use common safety sense when taking them, you're likely to reap some fantastic phytochemical rewards—maybe not the first time, maybe not even the second. Perhaps you purchased an inferior product. Generic pharmaceuticals vary in quality, so we can certainly expect to encounter greater fluctuations in the quality of herbal supplements.

Don't give up. Try again. Remember, too, that this science of ours is part art, and each of us responds differently to different things. The amount of kava kava that calms me down, for example, may do nothing for you. Or it may send you into a sound slumber. Dosage recommendations, whether in this book or on a label, are just that—recommendations.

Fortunately, phytochemical "farmaceuticals," by no means risk-free, are eminently safer than their prescription kin, even in large amounts. Use your head, first; don't go headfirst. Now, let's see what each of Duke's Dozen does and does not do for you and your good health.

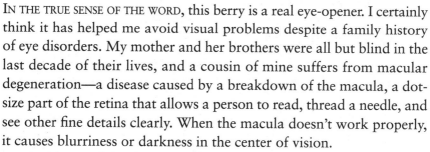

chapter three

Bilberry

LATIN NAME: *Vaccinium myrtillus*
FAMILY NAME: Ericaceae

IN THE TRUE SENSE OF THE WORD, this berry is a real eye-opener. I certainly think it has helped me avoid visual problems despite a family history of eye disorders. My mother and her brothers were all but blind in the last decade of their lives, and a cousin of mine suffers from macular degeneration—a disease caused by a breakdown of the macula, a dot-size part of the retina that allows a person to read, thread a needle, and see other fine details clearly. When the macula doesn't work properly, it causes blurriness or darkness in the center of vision.

I mentioned this family history of degenerative eye disease during a recent visit to my ophthalmologist. He checked and pronounced my retinas clean for now, but keeping my maculae in good shape is one of the reasons I take bilberry. It may not yet be on America's list of top 10 herbs, but it's on mine—and its popularity is growing as consumers discover the magic of bilberry's most important compounds, anthocyanosides. I believe bilberry can slow down visual degeneration, if not actually improve vision.

In addition, recently published studies have convinced me that bilberry—along with its cousins, the blueberry and cranberry—have even greater beneficial effects, both on specific ailments and overall good health.

What Bilberry Is and What It Can Do

The bilberry is an Old World equivalent of our North American blueberry. Like its relative, the bilberry is a food as well as a medicinal plant. As early as the sixteenth century, it was mixed with honey to create a syrup called rob, which was used to treat diarrhea.

About the size of a black currant, the bilberry is a round bluish fruit that grows on a small shrub that thrives in England, Scandinavia, and Siberia. The name bilberry is derived from the Danish, *bollebar*, meaning dark berry (and it is darker, at least inside, than our American blueberry). It is also known as Whortleberry, Black Whotles, and bleaberry. Some varieties are said to bear white fruits. These would be deficient in anthocyanosides, which are what give the bilberry its dark color.

Bilberries, when eaten fresh off the shrub, have a slightly acidic flavor. When cooked with sugar, they make an excellent preserve. In some European countries, the fruit is used for coloring wine.

Eyes-Wise in the West

Because it is more plentiful in Europe, bilberry is more widely accepted there than in North America. In fact, the berry is almost unheard of in the eastern United States and Canada. But plants rather similar to bilberry, such as dwarf bilberry, mountain blueberry, western blueberry, Mathers, and California huckleberry, are found farther west, from British Columbia south to Arizona, New Mexico, and Utah. My friend and colleague botanist Leigh Broadhurst tells me that bilberry is very popular in the West with an unlikely menagerie of users: sunbelt seniors in Tucson—sometimes with sunburnt eyes but mostly just getting on in years—and urban professionals in Seattle and Vancouver, likely trying to read in dimly lit coffee bars against the gray, rainy backdrop of the Pacific Northwest coastal climate. They must be using commercial imports, as I have no record of their being commercially grown in the West.

Bilberries have attained folk fame for treating vision disorders.

DR. DUKE'S NOTES

During World War II, the British gave bilberry products to Royal Air Force pilots to improve their night vision when they flew night missions.

Bilberry is what experts call a phytomedicine—that is, a healing substance rich in phytochemicals. Bilberry is a good source of phytochemicals, pigments called anthocyanins and related polyphenols. The pigments are molecules that give the bilberry and its cousins their deep red, blue, or purple colors.

The phytochemicals help stabilize the walls of capillaries, our smallest blood vessels. Like our joints and bones, the insides of our blood vessels are lined with connective tissue comprised of proteins, including collagen, elastin, and proteoglycan. The strength and flexibility of these connective tissues may be improved by bilberry. The result: the integrity of the eye's retina is maintained better or longer.

Traditional herbalists still recommend teas of bilberry fruit, combined with other herbs, to improve deteriorating vision. Bilberry leaves were a major component of antidiabetic teas in folk medicine, and while people still use them today, I can't endorse them because of their potential toxicity.

Bilberry is best-known today for improving vision disorders stemming from degeneration of the retina, the blood vessels which supply the retina, or both. These disorders include my own personal concern, macular degeneration, along with maculitis (an unspecified inflammation of the maculae), retinitis pigmentosa, poor night vision, and retinopathy. Bilberry may also help glaucoma and cataracts.

How Bilberry Can Help

Bilberry can be used to treat a variety of vision problems and can also be taken as a preventive measure against deteriorating vision. Here's a peek at some of its best-known applications:

Cataracts. Nearly 13 million Americans age 40 and older have cataracts, a clouding of the eye's lens. Cataracts become more common with age, possibly because the lens receives less nourishment as you get older. As a result, proteins in the eye begin to break down, causing the lens to become cloudy. Eventually, it can seem as if you are constantly looking through dense fog or haze.

In one impressive study, 48 out of 50 patients treated with bilberry extract and vitamin E arrested the progression of their cataracts. Italian researchers in the late 1980s found that a mixture of bilberry and vitamin E stopped cataract growth in 9 out of 10 cases. What's going on? In their useful book, *Prescription for Natural Healing*, James Balch, M.D., and his wife, Phyllis, a certified nutritional consultant, suggest that bilberry extracts contain bioflavonoids, which

 ## ALL IN THE FAMILY: CRANBERRY

I have six cranberry plants thriving in my herbal vineyard. As well they should. After all, cranberries, like blueberries, are an American original. Wild cranberries have been used by Native Americans for centuries and were quickly adopted by the pilgrims when they arrived in New England. Some native tribes boiled the dried cranberries and seasoned them with maple sugar. The English settlers found that this sweetened concoction made an excellent sauce for meats, including the traditional Thanksgiving turkey.

But the reason I keep a stash of cranberries in my garden has little to do with Thanksgiving—although I must admit it is certainly pleasing to stroll out into the vineyard and gather my own for this important holiday. Nor do I grow them for the esthetic beauty—although their pink blooms in early summer are appealing and their bright red berries are scintillating when ready for autumn harvest. The real reason I keep cranberries handy is much more pragmatic: They are a medicinal powerhouse.

How Cranberry Can Help

The cranberry has been used therapeutically since the seventeenth century for a number of conditions including stomach ailments, liver problems, vomiting, and appetite loss. Early New England sailors reportedly ate these vitamin C–rich berries to fend off scurvy.

The power of the cranberry is well-known in fighting urinary tract infections. The reason, evidently, is that the condensed tannins in cranberries prevent bacteria such as *E. coli*—the most common cause of infection—from attaching to the walls of the bladder and urethra. Since they can't attach themselves, they're more easily excreted with the urine and less likely to trigger symptoms.

Cranberries contain more than a dozen compounds such as flavonols, cat-

help remove harmful or undesirable chemicals from the retina.

Glaucoma. I have a genetic susceptibility to glaucoma. Often called the silent thief of sight, this disease, which usually strikes slowly, painlessly, and without warning, afflicts more than three million Americans. To understand how glaucoma robs vision, imagine that your eye is like a small sink. The faucet is a gland behind the iris

echins, and anthocyanins that may contribute to the relief of urinary tract infections. Because bilberry is rich in the same beneficial chemical compounds, it stands to reason that bilberry also may be helpful in treating urinary tract infections—and it's not quite so tart. Like bilberries, cranberries also have been shown to lower blood sugar. Cranberry juice has a reputation, deserved or not, for alleviating or preventing gout, perhaps by acidifying the urine. Cranberries might even have some Viagra-like effects, making it a potent weapon for those of you who suffer from urogenital problems previously known as frigidity and impotence.

How to Take It and How Much

Most cranberry drinks contain between 10 and 33 percent juice, though these beverages may be sweetened with other juices so the manufacturer can claim the product is 100 percent juice. So read the food label on the container carefully. I generally recommend drinking 3 ounces a day to prevent urinary tract infection, and up to 32 ounces daily as a treatment. Capsules containing 500 to 800 milligrams of dried cranberry powder are also available if you want to avoid sugar or sweeteners that are usually added to beverages. Two capsules are roughly the equivalent of 1 fluid ounce of cranberry juice. So to get the same preventive effect as the juice, you'd need to take six capsules daily.

Cautions

There are no known major side effects of cranberry, although drinking large amounts of the juice—three or four quarts daily—may trigger diarrhea. Cranberries should not be used in place of antibiotics during an acute urinary tract infection, but they may be used as an adjunct treatment.

that constantly produces fluid that bathes the eye. The drain has a mere 1/50-inch-wide opening. As you age, this drain tends to clog, and as a result, fluid builds up in the eye and increases pressure on the optic nerve. As the pressure increases, the nerve slowly begins to die and your peripheral (side) vision fades. Untreated, this condition eventually leads to almost total blindness.

Fortunately, after carefully checking my eyes, my ophthalmologist seems to think I may have outrun it—in other words, if I don't have it yet, the chances are good I won't get it at all. Bilberry, in combination with vitamin C and rutin, may help keep your eyes healthy. The vitamin C and rutin (found in pansies) can actually help lower the pressure within the eyes, and the compounds in bilberries called anthocyanosides retard the breakdown of the vitamin C, allowing it to do its job of protecting your eyes even better.

Macular degeneration. Macular degeneration may be linked to aging, since it most often strikes in later life. But what really triggers this malfunction is still a mystery. Family history, as in my case, is a prime suspect as are atherosclerosis (hardening of the arteries), dia-

 WHAT NEW RESEARCH TELLS US

Bilberry is best known for improving vision disorders, but new research suggests that it may be useful in treating a whole host of other health problems.

Recent studies have demonstrated bilberry's efficacy in treating circulatory complications due to diabetes or hypertension, bruising, capillary fragility, varicose veins, poor circulation, hemorrhoids, and Raynaud's disease.

Bilberry's beneficial effects may not stop there. In cell cultures, scientists have used anthocyanoside extracts to inhibit certain destructive enzymes—enzymes that degrade collagen and other connective tissue proteins. This type of degradation is a feature of atherosclerosis, pulmonary emphysema, multiple sclerosis, rheumatoid arthritis, and osteoarthritis. These conditions also benefit from higher levels of antioxidant protection, which bilberry and its cousin berries provide in abundance. So bilberry might help these conditions, too.

betes, and ultraviolet light. Bilberry can help slow down the degeneration process by preventing free radicals from damaging the macula and also by strengthening the capillaries in the retina.

Poor night vision. As you age, your eyes need more light to work properly. And in order to see well at night, your pupils have to get very large. Unfortunately, as you get older, your pupils simply don't dilate as well as they used to. Bilberry may help compensate for these changes. It is, for example, reported to significantly increase rhodopsin production within the eye. Rhodopsin is a purple pigment in the retinal rod cells—the cells used for night vision.

I mentioned my own worsening night vision to my ophthalmologist, who recommended glasses. But I will continue to supplement with fresh berries and bilberry capsules, and I will continue to enjoy those bilberry cousins, blueberries and cranberries, with my cereal in the morning, particularly if I have a predawn or postsunset drive ahead.

Retinopathy. A common complication of diabetes, retinopathy is a gradual visual deterioration caused by reduced circulation in the blood vessels that supply the retina. To compensate, the body creates new blood vessels in an effort to increase the blood supply to the eye, but these are typically weak and fragile—they leak and cause serious hemorrhaging in the eyes. Left unchecked, retinopathy can cause complete, irreversible blindness.

Bilberry helps strengthen blood vessels leading to the eye, improving circulation to the retina, which, in turn, enables it to function better. Studies have shown that 400 milligrams per day of standard bilberry extract reduced the tendency toward eye hemorrhaging in retinopathy patients, likely because bilberry may strengthen the blood vessels in the eye.

How to Take It and How Much

Bilberry fruit is available in several forms: fresh, unprocessed fruit, which can be hard to find, and bilberry extracts and capsules, which are more widely available. Personally, I'm hoping one day to harvest bilberries from my herbal vineyard, but for most people, I recommend a standardized product with known levels of anthocyano-

(continued on page 64)

ALL IN THE FAMILY: BLUEBERRY

I am a plant taxonomist by training, one of those botanists who studies the naming and identification of plants. Every plant has its own two-word scientific name in Latin, consisting first of the *genus*, followed by the *species*. Genus and species are the last two levels in the hierarchy of taxonomy, so every plant in a genus is closely related and every species is one of a kind. We taxonomists also like to tack on the name or initials of the scientist who first assigned the scientific name of the plant.

The generic name of the bilberry, *Vaccinium*, is the same as that of the blueberry and cranberry (see "All in the Family: Cranberry" on page 58). Think of them as cousins, members of the same large family. A closer pharmaceutical analogy is to think of them in the same way you think about generic prescription drugs. (These are the drugs beloved by your HMO due to their lower prices. Never mind how much could *really* be saved by prescribing the herbal alternative!) A generic prescription is one of several nearly identical forms of a drug, more or less interchangeable. The generic has the same basic actions, but it may be a little weaker or more impure, or a little stronger and purer, than the name brand drug it's knocking off.

I think of the bilberry, blueberry, and cranberry as generic phytomedicines. If anthocyanins are the active ingredients, then the bilberry seems to be the most potent. But if you can't get the "name brand" bilberry, you can substitute a "generic" blueberry or cranberry. And both blueberries and cranberries have beneficial health effects in their own right.

The Blueberry Murder

Believe it or not, the blueberry and I once got dragged into a murder trial in Maryland. I was called by both prosecution and defense lawyers to testify about the side effects that might result from drinking too much blueberry root tea. It seems that the defendant had allegedly imbibed both the tea and a considerable quantity of alcohol just before the murder.

At the time, I had dozens of facts at my fingertips about blueberry leaves and fruit. But if you'll pardon the pun, I had to dig around to learn more about the uses of the root. My own previous research uncovered Algonquian (Native American) use of the roots for urinary complaints. I further checked *Uses of Plants for the Past 500 Years*, which contains an account from Peter

Smith, author of *The Indian Doctor's Dispensary*, last printed back in 1901. According to Smith, blueberry root was the best of all camp medicines, used for everything from ague (fever) to childbirth, cholera, colic, cramps, epilepsy, hysteria, spasms, uretal inflammation, and hiccups. Smith even claimed that blueberry root stimulated the nervous system, although modern studies suggest otherwise. Other writers offered up similar broad claims for the root. A decoction was said to be good for diarrhea and other bowel ailments. Gargled, it was supposed to ease sore throats and mouths.

More telling for my purpose, however, was the suggestion that crushed roots and berries, when mixed in gin, were effective in treating dropsical afflictions (fluid retention or edema) and gravel (bladder and kidney stones). So there is, after all, an early precedent for mixing alcohol and blueberry root. I had to leave it to the lawyers, though, to figure out whether to use it to convict—or to dismiss the case. By the way, I don't use the roots myself, even in gin.

Blueberry Lore

Blueberry was very important to many Native Americans both as a food and a medicinal plant. Menominee Indians, for example, would dry the fruits like raisins for winter use and eat them mixed with dried corn, sweetened with maple sugar, as a special feast. The Iroquois reportedly mixed blueberries with their muffins, a culinary accomplishment celebrated again just this morning at my own breakfast table. A less appealing dish, at least to a near-vegetarian like myself, was a Chippewa combination of dried blueberries, moose fat, and deer tallow. Cooked long over a fire, it produced a blueberry pemmican said to last two years.

Native Americans also used blueberries for medicinal purposes—in fact, they may have influenced European thinking about the bilberry, which has been used as a food plant since time immemorial but as a medicinal plant only relatively recently, since the sixteenth century. The Ojibwa dried flowers of *Vaccinium angustifolum*, the lowbush blueberry, over hot coals and inhaled the fumes to treat "madness." The Ojibwa took the leaf decoction to "purify the blood," possibly a way to lower blood sugar. Algonquians used a blueberry leaf tea for colic, labor in childbirth, and following miscarriages. And

(continued)

various Native American tribes often added blueberry leaves to their smoking mixes.

What Blueberry Is and What It Can Do

The blueberry is a true-blue American food, one of the few food plants native to North America still found on American tables today (although it's notable that Native Americans used more than 1,000 food plants at the time Columbus arrived). It needs no introduction to most readers: It grows on low bushes in various parts of the United States and Canada, including Maine, and can be cultivated in all of the contiguous 48 states. Its round, sweet, blue-purple fruit is a favorite on cereal, in muffins, pancakes, and pies—although the best and most delicious way to eat them is fresh from the plant, picked in season.

Apart from its considerable culinary attributes, recent studies support my hunch that the blueberry shares medicinal attributes with its cousin the bilberry. Both blueberries and bilberries are noteworthy for their antioxidant capacity, but bilberry is by far the richer source of that miracle substance anthocyanoside.

Still, blueberries are known as the vision fruit in Japan, where they are reputed to help relieve eyestrain. And blueberries are emerging as the single most ferocious food in the supermarket for halting the forces that age you. In tests at the U.S. Department of Agriculture (USDA) Human Research Center on Aging at Tufts University in Boston, blueberries beat out 39 other common fruits and vegetables in antioxidant power—even such heavyweights as kale, strawberries, spinach, and broccoli. In fact, to get the same

sides. Extracts should be standardized to 36 percent anthocyanosides, and capsules to 25 percent anthocyanosides.

Effective doses used on patients in research studies are in the range of 320 to 480 milligrams of extract or up to two 400- to 500-milligram capsules per day. Lower doses of a 25 percent extract in the range of 80 to 160 milligrams three times per day have also been shown to be effective. Don't try these higher dosages on your own without consulting your doctor.

As a preventive measure, if you have access to unprocessed bilber-

amount of antioxidants in ½ cup of blueberries, you'd have to eat ¾ cup of strawberries, 1¼ cups of orange sections, or 2⅔ cups of corn.

Over time, as you probably well know, a diet rich in blueberries and other antioxidants can not only protect your vision but also protect your arteries, wrinkle-proof your skin, and strengthen your body's natural defenses. There's even some evidence that blueberries also prevent urinary tract infections and may help improve short-term memory.

The beneficial antioxidant activities of blueberries seem to be concentrated in the skin rather than the fruit. I suspect that cultivated blueberries have proportionately more water and fewer antioxidants than wild ones. So if I were looking for blueberries, I'd try to get hold of wild ones first, and then as a last resort, cultivated varieties.

How to Take It and How Much

Fresh blueberries are available year-round but are least expensive from May through September, when the supply comes from the United States and Canada. Look for berries that are dark blue, with a frosty bloom. Store fresh berries in your refrigerator for up to two weeks, and wash them just before you use them; otherwise, they'll get mushy.

Ronald Prior, Ph.D., head of the USDA Phytochemical Laboratory at Tufts University and the scientist who championed the secret power of blueberries, is so impressed with these azure nuggets that he now recommends adding ½ cup to your diet every day—a far cry from our current average intake of about 2½ cups a year!

ries, I recommend 20 to 60 grams of dried fruit or 100 to 300 grams of fresh fruit per day. If you are using bilberry in extract or capsule form, 80 to 100 milligrams three times per day is a reasonable dose.

Useful Combinations

Bilberry can be highly effective when taken in combination with other herbs, vitamins, and vitamin-rich foods.

Carrots. Don't overlook the familiar! I heartily subscribe to the maxim that carrots help our eyesight. Carrots are jam-packed with beta-carotene and other carotenoids, the precursors of vitamin A. These compounds, which make up the red, yellow, and orange pigments in plants, are converted into vitamin A in the body. Vitamin A is essential to make the visual pigment in our eyes. Carrot and carrot-based juices are helpful, but my data suggest that about half the beta-carotene is lost when you juice carrots, compared to just eating them as is or blending the whole carrot.

Rutin. Add rutin to your regimen as well. A suggested dose is 20 milligrams three times a day. Although buckwheat is popularly cited as a source of rutin, it's fairly common in lots of plants, also. I once calculated that one edible pansy flower would give you about 20 milligrams.

Vitamin C. Bilberry may work synergistically with vitamin C and rutin to lower the pressure within the eye characteristic of glaucoma. Some people respond well to 1 gram of vitamin C.

Caution: Contraindications, Interactions, and Side Effects

Bilberry fruit, extract, and capsules have no known interactions with commonly prescribed drugs and have no reported contraindications.

Pregnancy alert. Bilberry is reported to be safe to use during pregnancy and lactation, but I always recommend checking with your doctor.

Diarrhea. While there are no known side effects from using bilberry extracts in recommended dosages, too many fresh berries may cause diarrhea and/or a bluish black stool. On the other hand, dried bilberry fruits are recommended for checking diarrhea because they concentrate tannins and pectin.

Toxicity alert. Bilberry leaves can be poisonous if consumed over a long period of time or in great quantity. Commission E (a German panel of experts roughly equivalent to the U.S. Food and Drug Administration) does not sanction the bilberry leaf for therapeutic use. In animal studies, daily long-term administration of 1.5 grams of bilberry leaf per kilogram of body weight per day has been lethal. Although bilberry leaf teas are occasionally recommended, I suggest avoiding them.

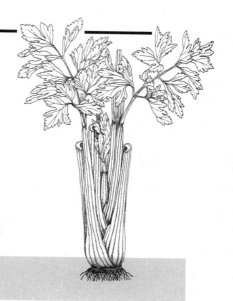

chapter four

Celery Seed

LATIN NAME: *Apium graveolens*
FAMILY NAME: Apiaceae

THE ONE MEDICINAL PLANT among Duke's Dozen that I take faithfully every day is the one I was initially the most skeptical about.

"The Crisis" is my name for a bout of gout, a condition I've endured for nearly two decades. I'd get attacks in my big toe so debilitatingly painful that words hardly do justice to the agony. I've suffered them enough over the years to know when they're all but certain to occur: after an injury, after a little alcohol-related overindulgence, or after I neglect to take my allopurinol, the pharmaceutical treatment of choice to prevent this condition.

The drug lowers the bloodstream's concentration of uric acid. At high levels, uric acid accumulates and then crystallizes in certain joints, typically the big toe. I so dread the pain these crystals cause that I took allopurinol faithfully almost every day for nearly 18 years.

Ever since I started taking celery seed, though, I've abandoned allopurinol. I simply no longer need it.

Celery is a good example of phytochemical medicine in action. For me, it's just as therapeutically effective as its man-made pharmaceutical rival—maybe more so. It's also safer. And you don't need a

(continued on page 70)

Going Toe-to-Toe with Gout

I was 49 when "the Crisis" (my term for a gout attack) struck for the first time. That summer, I was munching on fresh asparagus from my garden like it was going out of style. Asparagus is one of the many foods high in purines, substances that the body, courtesy of an enzyme called xanthine oxidase, converts into uric acid. Too much uric acid can lead to gout.

I awoke one morning to pain in my big toe so excruciating that I couldn't even stand the weight of a bed sheet on my foot. Imagine what it was like to put on a sock and attempt to walk. My doctor diagnosed the problem immediately and prescribed colchicine, a very heavy duty chemical (derived, incidentally, from the autumn crocus) that purges the crystals as it purges you. (Laxity is one side effect.)

For a while, I tried the dietary route, avoiding asparagus, organ meats, mushrooms, sardines, and other foods high in purines. All to no avail. Finally, another doctor suggested allopurinol (a pill a day for life for preventing gout) and indomethacin, a potent anti-inflammatory that stops gout attacks not prevented by allopurinol (or those that come on if you forget to take allopurinol). I didn't forget too often in the succeeding 18 years. In fact, I came to remember a few other things: that drinking a six-pack and forgetting my allopurinol (not necessarily in that order) brought on the Crisis the next day and that getting hurt also triggered an attack.

So on my merry way I went, studying plants as substitutes for pharmaceuticals and taking my man-made medication like a good little pain-fearing patient. Then one day I came across an advertisement for a phytochemical supplement that purportedly prevented gout. Celery seed extract, the ad claimed, was hypouricemic; it lowered uric acid.

I arched an eyebrow. I scoffed. I knew about celery seed. I've heard about its reputed medicinal properties. I had recorded everything known about the plant in my herbal archives. Sure, I'd read that it possessed some anti-inflammatory properties, but nowhere had I heard that it reduced uric acid. Itching for an argument and suspecting that he was motivated more by profit than science, I wrote to the man behind the ad, asking for more information about his research.

Imagine my surprise when I received copies of studies conducted in Australia and South Africa attesting to the anti-inflammatory qualities of celery seed extract. The science looked good. I was impressed. But how could I verify that it worked? I didn't have my own lab, and no other research in the world attested to the claims.

And then the dangerous idea dawned on me: I could serve as my own human guinea pig. No one, absolutely no one, is supposed to stop taking a drug without telling the prescribing physician. I beg you not to stop taking any medication on your own in favor of any herbal supplement advocated on these pages. Do as I say, not as I do.

Tossing aside everything I knew and believed about the advisability of discontinuing a medication, I stopped taking allopurinol. Instead, I swallowed, optimistically but hesitantly, four capsules of standardized celery seed extract. Then I braced myself. I was sure I'd wake up the next day to the oppressive load of the bed sheet on my big toe.

The next day, nothing. The day after that? Nothing still. For a week here at home in my herbal vineyard, I took celery seed extract. And my big toe was as happy as it could be. Coincidence? I didn't think so, but I couldn't be certain. I knew I'd find out soon, though. I had to leave for a week in Peru—a week of walking several miles a day through the rain forest, a week that inevitably would end with a parting ceremony filled with drink and dance. If ever there were a prescription for triggering the Crisis, this was it.

And so I went, armed with an ample supply of celery seed extract—and my anti-inflammatory medication, indomethacin, just in case. I toughed it out in the jungles all week long, and the gout held off. No problems. I didn't need the anti-inflammatory indomethacin.

Then on my last day there, we all convened at Tahuampa Bar, a thatch-roof refuge stilted over a tributary of the Amazon. We worked hard all week long and were ready to let our hair down.

It's a familiar scenario, one that I've been a part of many times before: lots of drinking, lots of over-vigorous dancing with guides who play great rancheros and salsa music. I recall an episode from years earlier in which spirited dancing to spirited music with spirituous Amazonian rum precipitated a splenetic attack of gout. Still, I didn't care. I was in the middle of an experiment.

(continued)

So this 67-year-old man took his celery seed extract, drank his potent Peruvian rum, danced—barefooted!—the dances of a 30-year-old, and threw caution to the wind. All evening long at the Tahuampa, we cut the rug and shook the mahogany floor. I remember, at one point, writhing to the beat with my partner, a masseuse who's a quarter or a third my age. We jumped up and down, then sideways, then up and down again, with me leaping higher and higher.

All of a sudden I felt an agonizing pain as I dropped down on my left foot. I thought I dislodged my hip from my pelvis. It hurt like hell. But, probably exceeding the legal limit for dancing, I kept on moving and finished out the song. Then, weary, hurting, and barely able to walk, I quietly absented myself and went to bed.

The next day greeted me with black-and-blue marks spanning some 15 inches from my left upper hip to below my buttock. It hurt. I could barely walk. But I tried not to show my pain. After all, in store for us that day were two hours on the Amazon, a long wait at Iquitos International Airport, and an even longer journey home. I didn't want to dampen anyone's fun, and complaining certainly wouldn't have put me out of my misery, although part of me wished someone would.

From the river, through Peru, and through long walks at the airports in Miami, Charlotte, and Baltimore, I was in agony all the way back—but not from gout. My big toe never let out a peep.

Knowing that traumatic injuries can conjure up the Crisis just as easily as a traumatic party, I fully expected a double-duty dose of gout pain. I anticipated it as a sentry awaits an imminent attack. At my side was a bottle of indomethacin, but I didn't reach for it. Instead, I took celery seed extract. I was, as I've said, in the middle of an experiment. In case an infection simmered

doctor's assistance or a discount prescription card to obtain it. You can swallow the seeds in standardized supplemental form. You can guzzle the reedy stalks as a juice or tonic, chew on them raw or relish celery's crunchy, flavorful presence in soups, salads, stews, and pot roasts. Try making a Bloody Mary with allopurinol. It won't work. And it won't taste very good, either.

near the damaged hip joint, I took some echinacea.

By all rights, I should have fallen over in agony somewhere between Miami and Charlotte. Certainly, I should have been causing an embarrassing scene in the aisle of the airplane somewhere over Virginia. But I didn't. I didn't feel very well, but I knew that gout wasn't part of my pain.

Finally back home, I took some turmeric and boswellin (along with celery seed), then crashed, anticipating that the Crisis would awaken me the next day. It didn't. In fact, I slept through my shift back to Eastern Standard Time, got up and performed my usual back exercises, walked out into my beautiful herbal vineyard, did some back stretches later on, took two more celery seed supplements, and felt pretty good. My wife was in Michigan, visiting our daughter. I was all alone—just me, the birds, and the other animals.

Well, that's not entirely true. The indomethacin was never far from ready reach. But I didn't need it—not so long as I had celery seed extract. As I walked around the garden, my limp grew less noticeable. I took it easy, but I was still using my brutally abused hip. By the end of the day, I concluded that I didn't even need to see the chiropractor or osteopath.

The next morning, I took more celery seed extract, felt even better, and continued to go about my business. Still no reason to take the indomethacin. Days wore on to weeks, weeks progressed to months. Before I knew it, Thanksgiving was at hand, then Christmas and New Year's and all the excesses that each holiday mandates. Throughout it all, the Crisis stayed away.

Should auld acquaintance be forgot and never brought to mind? I didn't forget my old acquaintance (gout) that holiday season, but I did the year after. And the year after that. With celery at my side, gout pain is just a ghost of grimaces past. Good riddance.

What Celery Seed Is and What It Can Do

If you ask Commission E (a German panel of experts roughly equivalent to the Federal Drug Administration), nothing about celery makes it worthy of recommendation. It's used only occasionally in folk medicine, according to the panel, mostly as a diuretic for kidney

HERB LORE AND MORE

Celery's light-green stalks seem so commonplace, so mundane that you might not suspect the plant boasts a long history of numerous therapeutic uses. Folk medicine practitioners dispensed various leaf preparations for cancerous ulcers, inflammatory tumors, herpes infections on the fingers (whitlows), and corns. Seed-based remedies were said to help breast and vulvar tumors. Celery juice could purportedly treat some forms of cancer in the eye and stomach, while a tea decocted from the seeds was said to help lumbago and rheumatism.

Other folk practitioners used the seeds against liver and spleen diseases, bronchitis, asthma, and flatulence. Indian medical experts believe the roots and leaves relieve colic, encourage excretion, and lessen tissue swelling from water retention. In Chinese medicine, the seeds are a standard treatment for dizziness, high blood pressure, calming the body, and regulating the menstrual cycle. The plant and its seeds have also been given to provoke menstruation and abortion. Celery's volatile oils do, in fact, induce uterine contractions and trigger menstrual flow. (Remember, an overdose of many, if not all, herbs and medicines can do the same or present problems for pregnant women. A former National Institutes of Health director has gone so far as to say that pregnant women and children should avoid all herbs. I cannot support such an extreme position.)

and bladder woes and as an ancillary supplement for rheumatism. The commission apparently didn't do the same homework I did and is thus a wee bit pessimistic.

I think Commission E is conservative in this respect. My own experience has convinced me that celery seed is an effective preventive for gout. For me, at least, no matter how much I tempt hyperuricemia, whether with an injury or a six-pack, celery seed seems to keep the Crisis at bay. Even three years into my experiment, my success could just be coincidence. Maybe I'm just one big 220-pound anecdote. But I doubt it. I think I'm on to something here.

How Celery Seed Can Help

Apart from gout, let's look at what other applications might work, too.

Arthritis and inflammation. Whether you suffer from gout or arthritis, you need to cool the fires. Celery seed is just what the doctor ordered for both conditions because of its myriad anti-inflammatory properties. Phytochemicals relieve pain and reduce water retention and tissue swelling.

Gas. In folk medicine, celery has a long-standing reputation as a "carminative," something that alleviates flatulence and the stomach pains associated with gas. I've received anecdotal accounts that relief comes rather quickly, too. According to other informal but informed reports, it also relieves indigestion, cramping, and heartburn.

Heart problems. Celery's active ingredients make it of potential

---

FROM MY SCIENCE NOTEBOOK

Celery is chock-full of substances that explain its healing properties. After I began to use myself as a guinea pig to ascertain its effect on gout, I turned to the U.S. Department of Agriculture databases for an assessment of its anti-inflammatory potential. I wasn't surprised to retrieve a list of some 25 anti-inflammatory compounds. Now we know why celery seed is an ingredient in some 60 British anti-inflammatory preparations.

Celery is also a good source of apigenin, which allows blood vessels to relax and dilate. This natural compound is just one of more than a dozen active ingredients that contribute to healthy blood pressure, either directly or by encouraging the body to excrete excess fluids—something Chinese medical practitioners have known for a long time. Natural calcium-channel blockers and heart rhythm stabilizers are among celery's myriad active ingredients, making the plant of potential value if you have arrhythmia (irregular heartbeat) or the chest pains of angina.

Little or no scientific research validates celery's other therapeutic uses. I can't confirm its effectiveness, either, but I can tell you that at least some of its phytochemical content explains folk uses against cystitis, kidney stones, and gallstones. Its essential oils possess some tranquilizing action, perhaps explaining its folklore use as a sedative.

value if you have arrhythmia or the chest pains of angina. With compounds that lower cholesterol and blood pressure, dilate arteries, thwart fluid retention and tissue swelling, normalize heart rhythm, and fight hardening of the arteries, I'd say it's a must-have medicinal for anyone concerned about cardiac health.

Hypertension. Celery contains apigenin, just one of about a dozen active ingredients that contribute to healthy blood pressure.

Science has confirmed celery's value from both clinical and experimental research. In one small study, 14 out of 16 men reduced their sphygmomanometer readings by drinking 40 milliliters of celery juice three times a day. Other lab investigations show that celery extract lowers blood pressure in dogs and rabbits; direct injections of an extract cut blood pressure significantly.

How to Take It and How Much

Until clinical trials compare celery seed extract, whole stalks of celery, and allopurinol, we'll never really know what the average person can rely on for freedom from gout or arthritis. Nor can we

 WHAT NEW RESEARCH TELLS US

We don't know if eating celery or taking it as a standardized supplement can improve blood fat profiles in people, but it appears to work for rats. In one study, scientists deliberately raised cholesterol levels in two groups of lab rodents by feeding them a high-fat diet for eight weeks. One group was then given regular supplements of a celery extract. Cholesterol profiles for the celery-swilling rats improved markedly, with triglycerides, low-density lipoprotein, and total cholesterol all dropping. In another experiment, a celery extract was given for 13 days to a group of rats genetically destined to have high cholesterol and to another group with normal blood fat profiles. The plant supplement prevented cholesterol increases among the genetically predetermined rodents, while blood fat readings among the other rats remained unchanged.

really know how much to take for heart-related help. One day, I hope, someone will conduct such research. Until then, I can only make guesses and tell you what works for me. You take it from there.

Supplements. At first, I took four capsules of standardized celery seed extract a day to keep the gout away. I later learned, though, that I could get by just as well on two daily capsules. The first capsules I took contained 800 milligrams of concentrated extract. Then I graduated to 500 milligram capsules, standardized to contain 450 milligrams of extract.

Food. My success bred further experimental daring and allowed me to discover that the "food farmacy" route works just as well. For two different two-week periods at home, I stopped taking supplements and relied on eating four stalks of celery a day. Gout still didn't put a crimp in my walk, even when I challenged myself with the six-pack test.

Right now, supplements remain the mainstay of my do-it-yourself gout treatment, but every once in a while the cheapskate in me emerges. If celery goes on sale at the grocery store, I'll buy bunches of bunches, juice and freeze most of it, but save some to eat.

Four stalks or two to four capsules a day may be enough to keep the cardiologist away, as well. Again, that's an estimation on my part.

Seeds. How else might you take celery seed? Some research reports success with an infusion tea made by mixing one-half to one teaspoon of celery seeds in a cup of hot water. Others suggest using ¾ teaspoon of crushed seeds per cup of water, taking 0.3 to 1.2

DR. DUKE'S RECIPES

Angelade

To enhance the phytochemical results in mild cases of hypertension, juice some garlic, onion, and tomato along with the celery. For more serious heart conditions and cardiovascular disease, I've concocted something I call "angelade." It's a juice made from angelica, carrots, celery, fennel, parsley, and parsnips. (Hawthorn makes a good addition for people with heart disease.) I'd like to think that angelade packs the calcium-channel-blocking punch of verapamil. I'll probably never know for sure, but I'll wager that it's safer than pharmaceutical calcium-channel blockers. It won't make your legs swell, it won't make you dizzy, and it won't give you a headache—all known possible side effects of these drugs.

milliliters of a 1:1 liquid extract three times a day.

For gas and gastric pain, chewing, but not swallowing, one teaspoon of celery seeds may help. For complete relief, you might have to chew on a second spoonful. I can't vouch for the remedy, however, because my experience in this regard is limited. I once tried it and found the seeds rather gritty. Right now, though, I'm getting hungry just thinking about sprinkling some seeds (maybe a tablespoon) on a piece or two of garlic-buttered toast.

Useful Combinations

I don't need anything else to keep the Crisis away. You might. For gout, arthritis, and help for heart problems, Mother Nature has stronger possibilities to which celery should serve as a companion. I'll mention the best.

For Outing Gout

Here are several useful combinations for getting gout out.

Cat's claw. In my pre-celery days, I once found myself caught with my pants down and my toe pain up. No pharmaceuticals on hand for help. Desperate for relief, I took a couple of pills that contained this herb, known for its ability to throw a bucket of water on inflammation. Nothing happened. So I took two more. Again, nothing. Two more pills later, still no relief. Neglecting the advice I always give others about ingesting too much of a medicinal herb, I swallowed a few more capsules. And a few more. When I had consumed a total of 12 capsules, I finally noticed some pain abatement. I'd never intentionally substitute *uño de gato*, as it's called, for celery in a case of the Crisis, but it could come in handy in a pinch.

Cherries. Science doesn't provide any reason for why the fruit might alleviate gout, but a friend of mine swears by black cherries, as do many other people. I once tried a juice made from tame and wild cherries, but it didn't impress me nearly as much as celery does, so count me out. Maybe the remedy will work for you. If you want to try, you'll need to eat about eight ounces of the fruit, canned or fresh.

Chiso. If you've given celery the chance it deserves but still double over with a painful big toe, try some chiso. This minty weed contains four different xanthine oxidase inhibitors that will help curb your body's production of uric acid. As a medication and a food, chiso is popular in the East. I like to put it in my mint teas.

Licorice. Get the real thing, not twisted sticks of the candy-counter impostor. True licorice raises blood pressure and lowers potassium levels in some people, so proceed cautiously. If you're not affected, my guess is that teaming up licorice and chiso will improve your overall antigout counterattack.

Turmeric. Another ingredient in Duke's Dozen, this Indian spice works via a different mechanism. The curcumin it contains deters certain pain-producing prostaglandins in the body. In high dosages, it also triggers the release of pain-easing cortisone from the adrenal glands. (See Chapter 15, Turmeric, for dosage information.)

Other foods. If you're caught without your celery, licorice, and cherries, other foods might get you out of that painful pinch. Eat more oats, olives, and pineapple. The first two are decent diuretics, while pineapple contains bromelain, an anti-inflammatory. Other herbs that might help harness gout pain include Devil's claw, stinging nettle, and willow.

Arthritis Aids

Pineapple is a smart pick if arthritis is your main complaint. Its bromelain helps the body get rid of two compounds implicated in the joint disease. Stinging nettle and willow, aspirin's original herbal form, are valuable here, too, though they might share the ulcer-inducing potential of aspirin and other nonsteroidal anti-inflammatory drugs. But you have a couple of other companions:

Ginger. Some 75 percent of the people with rheumatoid arthritis in one small long-term study felt better after they took ginger, in daily dosages ranging from three to seven grams. After more than two years, the relief persisted, and nobody ever felt any untoward effects.

Oregano. Oxidation apparently is part of the inflammatory process, and oregano contains some rather strong antioxidant chemicals. As research continues to affirm that antioxidants help to relieve both rheumatoid arthritis and osteoarthritis, I'd redouble my efforts to include oregano in both my food and my supplement regimen.

Red pepper. Maybe all of the pain perception is transferred from your joints to your tongue, but you gain a temporary respite from arthritic aches when you eat red pepper. It works topically, too. Capsaicin, the "hot" property in this plant, interferes with the transmission of pain impulses and encourages the body to release endorphins.

Other foods. Fortify your arthritis defense with Brazil nuts and sunflower seeds, both good food sources of the anti-inflammatory pain-relieving nutrient S-adenosyl-methionine, and rosemary, a good antioxidant partner to oregano.

A Hand for Your Heart

If you're looking for the premier phytochemical fix for cardiovascular health, especially as it relates to high blood pressure and high cholesterol, dog-ear this page and go straight to chapter 7 on garlic. Celery is pretty good against these two risk factors for heart disease, but garlic is one of the cornerstones of a natural treatment. Then turn to chapter 9 on hawthorn and similar heart herbs. Come on back when you're ready to finish your primer on celery seed.

Caution: Contraindications, Interactions, and Side Effects

I haven't experienced any. Nor did I knowingly fall victim to any of allopurinol's well-known side effects, which include skin reactions and eruptions, drowsiness, diarrhea, and nausea, not to mention the infamous "induction period," a month-long spate of time when you first start taking the drug during which gout attacks can actually increase. But many other people have.

I took allopurinol for almost 18 years, and I hope I'll be taking celery seed for the next 18 years to fairly compare its potential for side effects. In the meantime, I'll go with my instincts and predict that the natural is less likely to do harm than the unnatural. So far, 3 years have passed, and I haven't noticed any consequences. I doubt that it's much more dangerous than coffee, and I drank seven cups of coffee just as I wrote this section. I don't recommend that you drink seven cups, nor do I recommend that you take seven capsules of celery seed extract per day. Almost no one, though, should fear chomping on seven stalks of celery.

Photosensitivity. I once even tried to give myself a case of photodermatitis, which is sort of a bad sunburn caused by the interaction of ultraviolet rays and the presence of certain chemicals. Celery does contain compounds with this potential. Again using myself as a guinea pig, I expressed fresh celery juice on my arm, went outside, and exposed my wet flesh to the sun, trying, as I've done with the herb rue, to induce a phototoxic reaction and burn myself. But no burn!

You might be more sensitive, so don't try to replicate my dermatological experiment. The threat is real. Celery's phototoxic chemicals can increase some 200-fold during storage. One woman reportedly suffered a severe phototoxic reaction after ingesting celeriac, a close relative of celery, and then visiting a tanning parlor.

Allergy alert. Some extremely sensitive people have experienced a reaction after their skin simply brushed against some celery stems. Others have had anaphylactic reactions after eating the stems. (Let's not lose perspective, though. A hundred or so Americans die every year from anaphylactic reactions to eating nuts.) Additionally, for the few rare individuals with birch-celery syndrome, an allergy to birch or mugwort pollen, merely eating celery or its seeds can trigger an immediate reaction. Generally, though, the seed and the fruit have not provoked any side effects or toxicity problems.

Kidney problems. You may not have to avoid celery entirely if you have a renal disorder, but do be on the alert. The plant's oils can worsen kidney inflammation.

Pregnancy. If you're pregnant, you may want to wait until you've given birth to take celery therapeutically. In testing, its oils have encouraged uterine contractions.

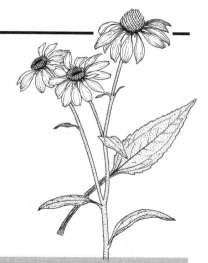

chapter five

Echinacea

LATIN NAME: *Echinacea angustifolia, E. pallida, E. purpurea*
FAMILY NAME: Asteraceae

YOU KNOW THAT famous advertising slogan: "Don't leave home without it"? That's how I feel about echinacea, America's most popular herbal medicine.

Echinacea is a powerhouse in the fight against colds and flu, as well as other viruses and infections. Not only has echinacea earned a slot among Duke's Dozen, second only to garlic, but it also rates a space in my travel bag, no matter where I go.

If I expect to shake hands after a speaking engagement, I want to know I'm defending myself from an energy-sapping bout of illness. The same goes if I'm visiting with the grandkids—or they with me. Colds and flu are highly contagious. Children average 6 to 10 colds a year, and adults 2 to 4, the National Institutes of Health reports. And influenza can strike up to 50 percent of a community when it makes its winter rounds.

But I haven't had a debilitating cold or flu in at least four years, since I started supplementing off and on with echinacea. Studies show it contains antiviral, antibacterial, and immune-boosting compounds.

In the winter of 1998, when my wife, Peg, and her sister got their flu shots, I declined to join them. Instead, I took standardized echinacea capsules and tinctures until the cold and flu seasons passed. Peg and her sister came down with some undiagnosed respiratory illness, maybe even the flu. (They may have already been infected when they got the shot, or picked up a different strain.) But I escaped the winter flu-less—not to mention cold-free.

This wonderful herb with the purple, daisylike flowers no doubt keeps me in the pink.

What Echinacea Is and What It Can Do

Echinacea, better known as purple coneflower, is native to the United States. Although it grows almost like a weed in my garden in Maryland—shooting to heights of two to three feet—it really is more at home in the Plains states. American Indians living there relied on it to heal just about everything, from toothaches to snakebites. It was a panacea for what ailed them.

Norman Grainger Bisset, professor of pharmacy at King's College of London and author of the excellent book *Herbal Drugs and Phytopharmaceuticals*, says that in the nineteenth century, echinacea was the most widely used plant drug in the United States. It was used to soothe sore throats, colds, bronchitis, and other infections. And it was applied topically to speed the healing of wounds and sores.

With the advent of synthetic pharmaceuticals in the twentieth century, echinacea lost favor for a while as a medicinal. But, in Germany, researchers have been looking at its immune-stimulating properties since the 1930s. Most studies on echinacea have been done in Germany and other parts of Europe, not in the plant's North American homeland. Until recent years, Americans have been slower than Europeans and Asians to embrace the value of medicinal herbs, even in their own backyards.

The positive results of the German studies, though, along with a renewed interest in nature's medicinals in general, are largely why consumers now scoop up echinacea products as wildly as the herb grows. In the United States, echinacea accounts for almost 10 percent of herbal sales.

It's no wonder our ancestors reached for echinacea. Although it grows like a weed, it is pretty. In spring, it puts out little rosettes of leaves close to the ground. Then, the stem reaches up to flower in late June and July, and sometimes until the first heavy frost. Some herbalists pick it after it flowers, while others say it's best harvested in the fall. But harvest they do, to satisfy an ever-growing clamor for echinacea products. More and more, stories abound in the United States and abroad about echinacea's preventive and healing abilities.

There have been a few negative reports, too. Some researchers dispute echinacea's preventive powers. But I say that any product this widely used is bound to take a few hits. The positive reports are overwhelmingly in this herb's corner. And so am I.

 ## HERB LORE AND MORE

Although it's been researched more widely in Europe, the purple coneflower is a native American, growing most abundantly in the Plains states. Native Americans likely were aware of its medicinal value long before early colonists stumbled upon this purple-flowered herb and its relatives *E. angustifolia* and *E. pallida*.

Daniel E. Moerman, Ph.D., professor of anthropology at the University of Michigan, has compiled a super database on the Native American uses of medicinal plants. I draw on his research for the following:

The Comanches made a decoction of the root to soothe sore throats and held the root against their teeth to ease toothaches. Chewing on the herb does cause a temporary numbness that may have proved helpful. The Blackfoot tribe also used angustifolia this way.

The Cheyennes relied on an infusion of the powdered angustifolia leaves and roots as a wash for painful necks and sore mouth, gums, and throat. They also used it to stimulate saliva.

The Dakotas believed the juice from echinacea soothed burns when applied to the skin. They used the plant as an antidote for venomous snake bites and other poisons. They applied poultices to reduce mumps. The tribe even used the plants in smoke treatments for horses with distemper.

The Lakotas chewed on the roots to ease tonsillitis and chomped on the plants to quell upset stomach and toothache.

Ounce of Prevention, Pound of Cure, or Both?

Much of the research has focused on the herb's strength at ousting colds and flu, when taken at the start of symptoms. Some studies show it also helps prevent viruses. Germany's Commission E (a panel of experts roughly equivalent to the U.S. Food and Drug Administration), has approved purpurea and angustifolia (and the roots of pallida, somehow disapproving of that herb itself) for treatment of colds, flu, and other upper-respiratory infections, such as bronchitis. One German researcher further reports that in a retrospective study of 1,280 children with bronchitis, those treated with juice made from echinacea recovered faster than those treated with antibiotics.

Whether echinacea is preventive has been more controversial, especially in the United States. A study out of Bastyr University in Seattle in 1999 indicated that people who took echinacea over six months had more symptoms of respiratory infection than those who took a placebo, according to one newspaper report.

Most researchers discourage its use for six months or longer anyhow. Many herbalists also believe the herb shouldn't be used year-round or for any long periods, because our immune systems may become resistant to it. I take echinacea only at the first signs of illness or when I know I'll be near crowds, or when there's a bad virus going around, but I believe it is beneficial in both prevention and healing. I'm still undecided about whether relying on it chronically challenges immunity, but I'm convinced echinacea gives me an edge.

Commission E also praises some echinacea for treatment of urinary tract infections and, topically, for wounds and other sores. Some research suggests it also may be helpful against other viruses, such as genital herpes, cold sores, sinusitis, and HIV/AIDS, and bacterial infections, such as pneumonia, sties, and streptococcal pharyngitis.

Sparring Over Species

Of the nine species of echinacea, three are most common, most studied, and most prescribed. They are E. purpurea and its close relatives, E. pallida and E. angustifolia.

I think I can tell the plants apart until they are reduced to tincture or powder. I have grown both angustifolia (whose leaves are narrow) and purpurea (whose leaves are wider and saw-toothed).

Studies show each of the common species contains a trio of key active ingredients: caffeic acid, cichoric acid (sometimes spelled chicoric), and echinacoside. Along with dozens of other phytochemicals, they fuel echinacea's antiviral, antibacterial, and immunity-enhancing reputation. Recent studies show that cichoric acid, in particular, exhibits many promising bioactivities.

A bit of sparring has arisen over which species is best. The truth is, we don't know. At least, not yet, and though the sparring partners each claim to have the best species, they haven't convinced me. Early chemical and pharmacological studies did not distinguish between species or plant parts. Some of the early work actually was done on a species called wild quinine.

No "voucher specimens" are on deposit in major herbaria for many of the critical studies. (We botanists relish voucher specimens for our research—they're pressed, dried, and mounted species of plants that we have studied.) Without such specimens, I can't tell whether a study was done on *E. angustifolia*, *E. pallida*, *E. purpurea* or black-eyed Susan, parthenium, chicory, or dandelion. And some chemists don't know the difference.

Still, I don't worry about which species I'm buying. I think all echinaceas have immune-boosting activities. Unlike man-made pharmaceuticals, nature's medicinals contain dozens of ingredients that work together for our benefit.

While I generally supplement, I can test the effectiveness of an actual plant simply by tasting it. Chewing on echinacea numbs the tongue temporarily. It's a harmless but sure sign of one group of active compounds called alkylamines. That's also the way "wildcrafters" judge the herb's potency in the woods. Some angustifolia from the Minnesota prairies has more zing than others I've sampled, but I'd be happy with any echinacea that makes my tongue go numb when I bite the plant in the field.

> ## DR. DUKE'S NOTES
>
> *You can buy cough drops, juice, soup, and even potato chips that contain echinacea. They probably won't help you get over a cold or flu, though. The dosages aren't standardized and are minuscule, at best.*

How Echinacea Can Help

The list of conditions that benefit from echinacea grows longer every day. In Germany, some researchers are even injecting the expressed juice of the plants for treatment of colds and flu—not a method I recommend. But I do suggest echinacea for the following:

Colds. You know the symptoms: coughing, sneezing, sore throat, runny nose. The National Institutes of Health calls the cold "probably the most common illness known." The more than 200 viruses that cause colds are easily spread, especially in enclosed environments with lots of people. Think school, day care, the office. Kids get 'em the most—and they love to share.

Just shake the hand of someone with a cold, put your hand to your eyes or nose, and you may come down with the virus yourself. Cold viruses can be breathed in when someone sneezes, and the particles can even float around in the air for a while.

Symptoms might be signs that our bodies are fighting back, the National Institutes of Health (NIH) says. Infected cells in the nose send out signals for disease-fighting white blood cells to get to work. Immune-system chemicals inflame the membranes in our noses and create fluids and mucus.

About 35 percent of the colds adults suffer are caused by rhinoviruses—from the Greek *rhin*, meaning nose—says the NIH. Usually, colds are mild and gone in a week or two. Other viruses, such as the respiratory syncytial virus, produce mild infections in adults but can cause more serious respiratory problems in children and the elderly. As many as half of all adult colds are believed to be caused by viruses that have not been identified, the NIH says.

Some studies show that immunity-enhancing compounds in echinacea lessen your chances of landing a cold—or its landing you. Scientists don't fully understand how echinacea stimulates immunity. Some think it increases properdin, a compound in the body that alerts the immune system to send out disease-fighting white blood cells. But there are many other mechanisms.

One preliminary study out of the University of Florida at Gainesville, in 1999, showed that echinacea stimulated the white blood cells of 10 healthy men who supplemented for four days. Nutritional sci-

Echinacea's medicinal power is threefold: It fights viruses and bacteria and enhances immunity. Active ingredients in the flowers, roots, and rhizomes appear to work together to prevent infection and promote healing.

At least three phytochemicals in echinacea are believed to be effective: caffeic acid, echinacoside, and cichoric (or chicoric) acid. All have antiviral activities (as do a dozen other compounds in echinacea).

Researchers are still trying to learn just how echinacea boosts immunity. Michael T. Murray, N.D., naturopathic physician and author of Natural Alternatives to Over-the-Counter and Prescription Drugs, says the herb raises levels of properdin, a natural compound in our bodies. Properdin tells the immune system to block viruses and bacteria by sending out infection-fighting white blood cells.

Scientists think echinacea's root extracts, in particular, may act like interferon, our bodies' own antiviral compound, says Norman Graninger Bisset, professor of pharmacy at King's College of London and author of Herbal Drugs and Phytopharmaceuticals. The roots may carry specific antiviral activity against flu, herpes, and other viruses, he says. Others say echinacea stimulates the body to make more interferon, along with interleukins and tumor necrosis factor, signaling molecules that enhance immune response.

The herb's immune-boosting activity may possibly stimulate some progressive conditions, including HIV/AIDS, some researchers believe. Recently, however, research has shown that cichoric acid may have anti-integrase activities. Integrase is what HIV uses to infiltrate the DNA. So, echinacea may actually help fight HIV/AIDS, as well as other viruses.

entist Susan Percival of the University of Florida's Institute of Food, who led the research, cautioned that her work did not support the regular use of echinacea in the absence of cold symptoms.

It might be best to reach for echinacea only when colds are all around you—or at the first hint of symptoms. Echinacea's cold-busting abilities are better documented, at least for now. In one double-blind study in Germany of 180 cold patients, those treated with high-dose echinacea recovered faster than those taking lower doses or a placebo.

If you take it often, some herbalists say, at least cycle on and off the herb. In an interview in *Complementary Medicine for Physicians*,

(continued on page 90)

WHAT NEW RESEARCH TELLS US

Here's a rundown of the research-in-progress and what it may tell us about the future of echinacea and healing. Remember, though, that this is cutting-edge research, and more confirming studies are needed.

Sun-damaged skin. Researchers have noted that several compounds in echinacea, including cichoric acid, caffeic acid, chlorogenic acid, rutin, and echinacoside, lessen the destruction of collagen, which gives our skin its elasticity. Maybe echinacea will play a role in helping to prevent skin damage from sun. Eric Yarnell, N.D., says test-tube studies indicate phytochemicals in echinacea might also protect against ultraviolet damage—and that we might soon see it in a sunburn ointment.

Lyme disease. The leaf and root of purple coneflower are mildly antibacterial. Could the herb help fight the bacteria (*Borrelia burgdorferi*) carried by the deer tick? It may be something to watch for, although a boosted immune system might fight better.

A few years ago, I dodged a possible case of Lyme disease, and I think echinacea may have helped. I had been filming with a television crew in my herbal vineyard and thought we would be outdoors only briefly. A few minutes turned into two hours. Although I usually wear an herbal bug repellent, I was unprepared and unprotected.

Slapping my leg at what felt like an insect bite, I saw nothing there and forgot about it. Deer ticks are so small that until they are engorged, I can't see them without my glasses. The next day, I developed the characteristic bull's-eye—redness around a white halo and a red mark in the center—that typically follows a bite by a deer tick carrying *Borrelia burgdorferi*, the bacteria that causes Lyme disease.

Because it was the weekend, and my HMO doesn't treat anything but emergencies on weekends, I immediately began my own home-prescribed regimen of standardized echinacea capsules, along with garlic, another immune stimulant. I didn't want to develop arthritis, an unpleasant possibility when Lyme disease goes untreated. At Peg's urging, I visited a physician the following Tuesday; he prescribed doxycycline, a synthetic antibiotic.

Although I never had a blood test to confirm that I was bitten by a tick that carried Lyme disease, I didn't come down with any other symptoms, including the dreaded joint pain and inflammation of arthritis. I like to think that echinacea, along with garlic and the antibiotic, may have helped me beat the disease and its potential complications, such as arthritis and stiff neck, temporary paralysis of facial muscles, and other neurological symptoms. And the three days I gained by starting with my herbal antibiotic before doxycycline may have been critical. We'll never really know.

Hepatitis C. This liver infection is caused by the viral hepatitis. A 1998 report in *Herbs for Health* reveals that British-trained phytotherapist Amanda McQuade Crawford, founding member of the American Herbalists Guild, founder and director of the National College of Phytotherapy in New Mexico, and another grande dame of herbalism in the western United States, has had success treating viral hepatitis using a diuretic and mild antiviral. For one of her patients, Crawford combined the diuretic Lasix with silymarin, the concentrated active lignans in milk thistle, and dandelion. Within three months, her patient no longer needed the Lasix. Furthermore, tests showed improved liver enzymes and viral load, which means fewer counts of virus per unit measured.

Based on evidence showing that the flowers of echinacea are an excellent source of cichoric acid, which may slow reproduction of viruses, I would add echinacea to my milk thistle if I had viral hepatitis.

Sinusitis. In "The Botanical Approach to Chronic Sinusitis" published in 1998 in *Alternative and Complementary Therapies*, Dr. Yarnell says echinacea's immunologic effects are likely to help many sinus sufferers. His sinusitis formula includes echinacea as its top ingredient. My colleague Steven Morris, N.D., a naturopathic physician practicing in Washington state, recently told me about a patient under his care for chronic sinusitis, inflammation of the sinuses caused by infection or allergy. The patient had multiple sinus surgeries, Dr. Morris says, and more than 10 courses of antibiotics in five years. Using his "Sinus Survival" protocol, the patient had not used antibiotics in nine months and, instead, supplemented with *E. angustifolia*. The regimen included 300 milligrams liquid of the root, along with the plants Oregon grape, milk vetch, privet, and Chinese magnolia.

Yeast infections. German researcher Rudolf Bauer reports that echinacea may prove effective at treating vaginal yeast infections. In one study, women who used econazole nitrate, the standard remedy, had a 61 percent rate of recurrence. The rate dropped to 5 to 16 percent, Bauer reports, when echinacea was used along with the standard drug.

M.E. O'Brien, M.D., suggests starting echinacea in October, at the beginning of cold and flu season, and taking a few days off every two to three weeks.

Flu. A variety of influenza viruses causes this respiratory infection. Unlike colds, symptoms begin abruptly and may include headache, chills, body aches, and fever. Coldlike symptoms, such as nasal congestion and sore throat, follow. Most people recover within a week but still feel tired after other symptoms have passed. Young children, the elderly, and people with compromised immunities are at risk for more serious illness, such as pneumonia, the NIH says.

Like colds, flu spreads rapidly from person to person, especially from coughing and sneezing. Often, it pops up where there are lots of school-age children. The highest incidence of flu is in 5- to 14-year-olds.

The traditional prescription for flu is similar to that for colds: rest, fluids, and aspirin or acetaminophen. The synthetic drug rimantadine may be effective if it's used within 48 hours after symptoms begin.

Although people often ask their doctors to prescribe an antibiotic, these drugs are not a treatment for flu or viral colds. Such dependence on these pharmaceuticals has created a danger in our world: Antibiotics may one day be ineffective against the bacteria they were designed to destroy.

The vaccine for flu prevention that is widely available is made from killed viruses. It must be given six to eight weeks before flu season to prevent infection. But influenza is always changing. You may be protected against one strain and still come down with another. In flu season, I boost my immunity with standardized echinacea. Some may question the preventive effects, but I believe echinacea protects me from infection.

Germany's Commission E has approved certain species of echinacea for treatment of flu, based on years of European research. One study of 180 people with flu showed that echinacea extract significantly reduced symptoms.

As with colds, scientists don't know specifically how echinacea works against flu. Not only does it likely raise properdin to produce disease-fighting white blood cells, but some researchers say it stimulates immunity by way of interferon and interleukins.

I suspect echinacea's success lies in the synergy of its many active ingredients, working in many channels and stimulating the immune system in many ways.

HIV/AIDS. The National Institutes of Health says nearly 900,000 Americans may suffer from HIV, the virus that causes AIDS. The virus kills or cripples the immune system's T-cells, leaving victims unable to fight infections and certain cancers. There is no cure.

Standard treatment includes costly drug "cocktails" that work in combination. AZT interrupts early stages of virus replication. Other drugs called protease inhibitors interrupt the virus at later stages. The regimens are tough to stick with. Some studies indicate that when the drugs are stopped, patients show antibodies in their blood—a sign the virus has not been beaten, only stalled.

The research to find a cure continues. But some of the most exciting reports I've seen have focused on cichoric acid, a compound in echinacea, as a potential treatment for HIV. Only a couple of years ago, most herbalists, including myself, advised against supplementing with echinacea for patients with HIV. Some researchers say the herb stimulates the virus, as well as immunity. But in 1996, *U.S. Chemical and Engineering News* praised synthetic cichoric acid for its integrase-blocking—and presumably antiretroviral—activities. The virus uses integrase to get into the DNA of cells.

> ### DR. DUKE'S NOTES
>
> *Purple coneflower, or echinacea, is also pretty to look at. It sprouts in the wild, but you can purchase it at your local nursery. Until the recent rage over its medicinal value, the plant was more commonly used as an ornamental in both Europe and the United States. Its popularity as an ornamental probably is increasing because of its newfound fame as a medicinal.*

Since then, I have learned that cichoric acid is abundant in the flowers of many echinacea species. It makes up as much as 3.1 percent of the plant's dry weight and is plentiful in the roots of purpurea, as well.

If I had HIV/AIDS, I would munch on the flowers of the purple coneflower, so far the best known source of cichoric acid, in addition to the drug cocktail treatments my doctor prescribed, if I could afford them.

Wounds and sores. Some studies show that echinacea has topical healing qualities, too. The herb has antibacterial and antiseptic properties that may speed recovery. Commission E has approved some echinacea preparations topically for the treatment of various wounds and sores.

Eric Yarnell, N.D., a naturopathic physician in private practice in Sedona, Arizona, and a frequent writer for the journal *Alternative and Complementary Therapies*, mentions an array of topical uses in his article "Botanical Medicines for Dermatologic Conditions" published

 A CASE IN POINT

Lolen's Story

Lolen D., a full-time college student living in Virginia, has relied on echinacea for protection from colds and flu for about four years. She became curious about it after a friend told her about an article she'd read on the 10 best herbs for winter; echinacea was among them. Lolen already was a believer in the value of a handful of other herbs as well as daily multiple-vitamin supplements. So she added echinacea to her medicine cabinet.

For three winters, Lolen used the 200-milligram capsules every now and then—"whenever I'd start to feel under the weather . . . tired, run-down, sniffly," she says.

Looking back after each season, she realized she was getting sick less often. So, in the winter of 1998, Lolen tried an experiment. She used echinacea more diligently, along with vitamin C and zinc. "This is the first time I took it religiously," says the 30-year-old.

At the onset of cold or flu symptoms, Lolen reached for her trio: 500 milligrams of vitamin C three times daily; zinc lozenges to chew on throughout the day; and 200 milligrams of echinacea three times a day, for two weeks at a time. She had read a lot about echinacea and knew that taking it every day might lessen its immunity-enhancing effects.

That winter, Lolen zipped through her semester of studies without a cold or flu. "It's proven itself this year," she says, noting that she stays with a brand she trusts, purchased through a health food and vitamin store.

Now, Lolen tells her friends about what works for her—echinacea, zinc, and vitamin C. "That," she says, "seems to be the winning combination."

in 1999 in *Alternative and Complementary Therapies*. He says European research shows it soothes many skin conditions, including burns, ulcers, varicosities, dermatitis, herpes simplex, and psoriasis.

Historically, echinacea has been applied to heal carbuncles, boils, bedsores, cellulitis, folliculitis, gangrene, smallpox, stings, and the blistery rash of chickenpox. I don't think our Native American forerunners were foolhardy. Echinacea proved itself to them long before we started packaging it in colorful boxes and bottles.

How to Take It and How Much

Generally, I don't use the plant or its extracts from my garden, because I want to be sure I'm getting the same amount of active ingredients every time. Besides, my plants are too pretty and too much trouble to sacrifice, when I have standardized extracts and tinctures in the house.

E. purpurea and related species are most commonly available in tinctures, capsules, and teas. Often when I supplement, I use both tinctures and capsules. When I shop for a supplement, I look for a product that's standardized. I tell people to find a brand they trust and stick with it, because a wide range of grades is on the market. (There's a lot of money to be made, now that echinacea has grown famous. And some of the wild populations are threatened by greedy over-collecting.)

Here are some recommendations for use, based on my experience.

Colds and flu. Buy standardized capsules and follow label directions, either at the start of the cold and flu season or as symptoms appear. You may want to add a standardized tincture to your regimen to get the full benefit from echinacea's active ingredients, especially if you're in a high-risk environment. Varro E. Tyler, Ph.D., Sc.D., professor emeritus of pharmacognosy at Purdue University, prefers extracts to capsules. As Dr. Wallace J. Murray, Ph.D., associate professor of pharmacy at the University of Nebraska Medical Center, reminds us in a new book co-edited with Lucinda G. Miller, Pharm.D., *Herbal Medicinals—A Clinician's Guide*, 1998, Dr. Tyler recommends swishing the tincture in your mouth for a while before swallowing, to stimulate the oral lymphatic system.

HIV/AIDS. Herbalists sometimes warn against taking echinacea every day, because our bodies may get used to it. If I had HIV, I would reach for standardized echinacea capsules daily for a week or two, then stop and start again. And I'd be eating those petals for their cichoric acid, too, maybe even daily. I also recommend a tea, using 5 teaspoons dried echinacea per cup boiling water, two or three times a day.

Another option: Add a dropperful of tincture to juice and drink it several times a day. Herbalists used to discourage HIV patients from taking echinacea, but new research shows cichoric acid may help keep the virus from infiltrating DNA. We have to rethink our positions as new evidence emerges, especially with life-threatening diseases such as HIV.

Wounds and sores. Dr. Yarnell, writing in *Alternative and Complementary Therapies*, suggests making a compress using the plant extract and applying it directly to the skin, changing it several times daily. You can mix an extract with a cream or lotion and apply it that way, also. Or whip up your own ointment by adding the extract to an oily or waxy salve or unguent, and apply it several times a day, Dr. Yarnell says. A poultice may be made with the fresh herb and placed on the skin. I would simply open a capsule and apply the powder to my wound.

Useful Combinations

Echinacea may be especially helpful when combined with other medicinal herbs or traditional methods of prevention and treatment.

Garlic. I often combine this personal favorite for boosting immunity with echinacea when I want a megadose of protection against colds, flu, or other viral infections or bacteria. I believe this potent combo of immunity boosters has helped me stave off Lyme disease, perhaps even more than once.

Goldenseal. You might add this immunity-enhancing herb to your cold and flu arsenal. As I mention in *The Green Pharmacy*, goldenseal contains berberine, which also activates those disease-fighting white blood cells. It has antiseptic activity, too.

Hand washing. Frequently washing your hands is one of the best ways to prevent colds and flu. You can pick up the germs by putting a hand to your eyes, nose, or mouth after touching a person or surface where the germs are.

Rest. Try not to burn the midnight oil, especially in cold or flu season. Fatigue dampens immunity and makes you more prone to infection. Can't sleep? Sip some chamomile tea before bedtime. Echinacea is one of the safest medicinals, natural or synthetic.

Zinc. Many over-the-counter cold remedies tout the zinc-echinacea combination. The addition of this mineral may help heighten immunity. You also can get zinc in your diet. Sources include oysters, wheat germ, parsley, collards, brussels sprouts, cucumbers, string beans, and spinach. (Maybe that's why Popeye and spinach got along so well.) Try adding vitamin C supplements to help reduce the severity and length of colds.

Caution: Contraindications, Interactions, and Side Effects

Commission E reports no side effects or interactions with other drugs. However, a lot of press was directed against echinacea in 1998, probably stemming in part from a misinterpretation of the literature on pyrollizidine alkaloids. The press warned about potential liver damage when using echinacea for only a short time. I know of no studies showing that echinacea damages the liver. It may take a couple of years to undo the damage from that erroneous report, however.

But there are some cautions you should keep in mind before taking echinacea.

How often is too often? Some experts say echinacea shouldn't be used steadily for more than two to six weeks. Commission E says no more than eight weeks.

Pregnancy. Other sources suggest avoiding it altogether if you are pregnant or hypersensitive.

Allergy alert. One report out of Australia connects echinacea to serious allergic reactions. The Australian Adverse Reactions Bulletin tallied 36 reports to general practitioners of adverse reactions, from 1990 to 1999. One-third related to asthma or allergies. That compares to 24 adverse reports for evening primrose, 13 for garlic, and 10 for ginkgo. Australian botanical researcher Andrew Pengelly says the most widely used herbs are bound to produce the greatest number of reports. Most of the 36 cases, he notes, subsided without treatment and came from as many as 200 million doses a year.

HIV/AIDS caution. Up until about two years ago, echinacea was contraindicated for anyone with HIV/AIDS, because it was believed to stimulate the virus as well as the immune system. Commission E cautions that echinacea should not be used by anyone with an autoimmune disorder, including HIV/AIDS, multiple sclerosis, tuberculosis, collagenosis, and leukosis. I believe the discovery of cichoric acid's potential demonstrates that we need to reconsider its usefulness in helping to treat HIV/AIDS. Studies showing it activates the virus involved megadoses, not those found in standard formulas. But the final word is still out; caution is key.

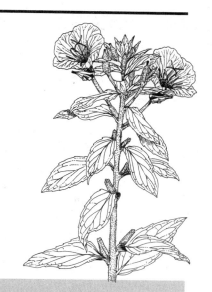

chapter six

Evening Primrose

LATIN NAME: *Oenothera biennis*
FAMILY NAME: Onagraceae

DURING A RECENT TRIP to Costa Rica, I overheard two women, both pharmacists, discussing the effectiveness of evening primrose oil for premenstrual syndrome (PMS).

One said she faithfully took one capsule of evening primrose oil (EPO) daily for about two weeks every month and then upped the dosage to four capsules daily a week before menstruation. She stayed on the quadruple dose until her period was over. Her herbal regimen worked so well that she'd passed it along to five female co-workers.

"We've been working together so long that our periods are almost synchronized," she said. "I hate to imagine what would happen without evening primrose oil. Think of all of us with PMS at the same time each month!"

Women who suffer from premenstrual syndrome endure varying degrees of monthly misery. They report such symptoms as water retention, breast soreness, cramping, diarrhea, irritability, chronic headaches, and tension.

Up to 50 percent of menstruating women experience some symptoms of PMS, sometimes severe enough to be temporarily debilitating. Experts think the cause is linked to hormonal fluctuations and the body's inability to properly metabolize fatty acids.

As a botanist who's done a lot of research on evening primrose, I'm convinced it's an effective, natural premenstrual syndrome reliever. At my lectures, I frequently encourage women to try it, and I've shown many of them—including my own daughter—how to gather and chew evening primrose seeds just as Native American women once did.

Doctors in Great Britain, where evening primrose is approved for treating PMS and other health conditions, agree with me. There, the firm Scotia Pharmaceuticals has invested $80 million in researching evening primrose.

But here in the United States, a surprising number of women still don't know that this highly effective herbal remedy is within reach, even though it's readily available in health food stores. I blame the Food and Drug Administration (FDA), which prohibits labeling evening primrose as a natural PMS helper because it's still not an approved remedy in this country.

Instead of discounting British research studies supporting evening primrose, the FDA should take steps to recognize what many herb experts already know: Evening primrose works, and it's at least as safe as coffee.

In the meantime, I'm doing my part to get the word out. Even if you're not a PMS sufferer, evening primrose can be helpful for conditions that affect men and women alike. It's rich in gamma-linolenic acid (GLA), a substance useful in treating a number of conditions including endometriosis, autoimmune disorders, benign prostatic hypertrophy, eczema, diabetes, and migraines.

What Evening Primrose Is and What It Can Do

Sweet-smelling evening primrose is no relation to the primrose that bedecks your border garden. That garden primrose hails from the *Primula* family, a different botanical clan altogether. The herb variety is a biennial plant that grows from three to nine feet tall. It sometimes has woody stems. Its willow-shaped leaves may taste a bit peppery, and the root much more so. At twilight between June and October, the evening primrose unfolds its lovely lemon-colored (but short-lived) flowers, whose scintillating sweetness encourages pollination. By dawn, the blossoms start wilting, and new ones flower toward the following dusk.

This night bloomer is a native to North America, growing in meadows, fields, and along roadsides. Evening primrose flourishes in virtually all 48 states, maybe all 50. While it is generally considered a weed in the United States, evening primrose is planted as an ornamental flower in Europe.

Evening primrose oil is extracted from the seeds of the plant. Both the seeds and oil contain gamma-linolenic acid, but most people take this herb as an oil, generally in capsule form.

I place a lot of stock in the British research supporting evening primrose, but not everyone does. While I have great respect for the German Commission E (a panel of experts roughly equivalent to the U.S. Food and Drug Administration) and Varro E. Tyler, Ph.D., Sc.D., professor emeritus of pharmacognosy at Purdue University, neither ranks evening primrose or its cousins, borage and black currant, as highly as I do. Nor, sadly, does the FDA. I consider it *the* drug of choice for PMS.

How Evening Primrose Can Help

Evening primrose can ease a variety of conditions, especially those resulting from an imbalance of essential fatty acids, inflammation of the skin, or an immune deficiency.

Alcoholism. Studies suggest that EPO can help recovering alcoholics cope with withdrawal symptoms experienced during the first three weeks they stop drinking. Patients who take EPO may require fewer tranquilizers, and their livers may begin proper functioning more quickly. Research also shows, however, that the oil has no effect on preventing relapse.

Arteriosclerosis. When cholesterol, lipid, and calcium deposits line the arteries, causing them to harden, arteriosclerosis is the dangerous result. When combined with a low-cholesterol diet, EPO shows promise in reducing the risk of arteriosclerosis, probably because it contains anticlotting compounds.

Asthma. This disease causes wheezing and tightness in the bronchial airways. It's often triggered by an allergic reaction. People with asthma can breathe easier thanks to evening primrose leaves. They contain quercetin, a good remedy for asthma and hay fever sufferers alike.

Benign prostatic hypertrophy (BPH). Evening primrose works for men as well as women. When the prostate gland becomes inflamed and grows larger in aging men, it can cause numerous side effects including urinary difficulties and impotence. This condition, BPH, is also called noncancerous prostate enlargement. Research indicates that 50 percent of men have some degree of prostate enlargement by age 50. Further, at least 90 percent of all men 70 to 90 years old, by some estimates, must contend with BPH and its symptoms. Thirty zpercent of them undergo surgery. Doctors take matters of the prostate very seriously because prostate cancer is the second leading cause of death in men of all ages.

I bet my own prostate that herbs work better than prescribed medications or surgery to control prostate growth. (I really did. See chapter 14.) Science is showing I might be right. EPO was reported in the *Journal of Urology* to help prevent prostate problems because it acts as a powerful 5-alpha-reductase type II inhibitor, which helps reduce enlarged prostates. For my part, I'll continue taking EPO and saw palmetto to maintain my good prostate health. I'll also keep on adding the gritty, ground-up evening primrose seeds to my cornbread recipe as I've done for the last 15 years, off and on.

Depression. Tryptophan, a chemical compound found in evening primrose seed, may help to alleviate depression, perhaps as well as—and surely as safely as—the synthetic alternatives, including Prozac. Tryptophan is a precursor of brain serotonin, known for its mood-boosting effects.

Evening primroses are happy flowers. Just cultivating them tends to reduce stress and lift your spirits, and spending time outdoors in the sunshine also does wonders for your mental well-being.

Diabetes. People with diabetes may experience a condition called diabetic neuropathy, which can cause loss of feeling in their extremities. Naturopaths often prescribe evening primrose oil because it's rich in tryptophan, which helps stimulate the central nervous system. Much of EPO's tryptophan is lost during the oil-extraction process, though, so I'd recommend powdered seeds instead.

Eczema. Skin-soothing evening primrose oil is approved in the United Kingdom to treat eczema, a skin condition that causes inflammation, redness, itchiness, burning, and scabbing. Studies on laboratory animals have shown that the seed oil can reduce swelling. Research shows the oil's GLA can be effective when applied to other skin irritations such as dermatitis. I wouldn't hesitate to put a little EPO on a bug bite or rash, either.

For eczema, take the herb orally. Borage and black currant are

HERB LORE AND MORE

The evening primrose has a rich history as a folklore remedy amongst Native Americans. Dr. Daniel Moerman, Ph.D., a highly respected authority on the subject, says that Cherokee tribes often applied the hot root onto hemorrhoids and drank the tea to counteract obesity, which he terms "overfatness." Today, evening primrose oil is still occasionally used as a folk remedy for the same purpose.

Iroquois tribes are said to have used evening primrose as a dermatological salve for boils and skin eruptions, and naturopaths still prescribe the herbal oil to treat a variety of skin irritations.

also chock-full of GLA. They're available in capsule form and should be taken as directed by the manufacturer's instructions.

Endometriosis. When the membrane that lines the uterus becomes inflamed, low back and abdominal pain, constipation, and vaginal discharge may occur. The natural remedies guides I respect the most mention EPO as a treatment for this condition. One clinical trial shows that 90 percent of women treated with gamma-linolenic acid experienced improvement. While it's true that EPO's compounds promote good health in women, I still think of evening primrose oil more as an herbal medicine to address PMS than for treating endometriosis because there is much more research to support it.

High blood pressure. When blood pressure is higher than normal, the heart's workload is increased. My colleague David Horrobin, Ph.D., editor of the British journal *Medical Hypotheses*, who has written extensively about the nutritional and medical importance of GLA, reports that it is effective in lowering both cholesterol and blood pressure.

High cholesterol. Elevated blood cholesterol levels can increase your risk for heart disease. The GLA in evening primrose is reported to lower cholesterol levels. If I had high cholesterol, I'd eat a low-fat diet, quit smoking, and add EPO to my heart-healthy regimen.

HIV. The life expectancy of HIV patients more than doubled when GLA and omega-3 fatty acids were included in their diets, according to studies done by researchers in Tanzania. Both GLA and omega-3 fatty acids are essential to maintaining cell structure membranes and making hormonelike substances known as eicosanoids, which help regulate blood pressure, blood clot formation, blood lipids, and the immune response to injury and infection. The body can make all other fatty acids except for these two, which must come from the diet. After reviewing the medical literature, I wholeheartedly believe that GLA can be a potent treatment for autoimmune disorders, including HIV. If I had it, I'd take EPO for its GLA and add fish oil or flax seed oil (the vegetarian option) to my diet. Both are good sources of omega-3 fatty acids. I'd take EPO for another autoimmune disorder, Sjögren's syndrome, too.

Multiple sclerosis. Multiple sclerosis, or MS, is a chronic autoimmune inflammatory disease that affects the central nervous system, causing nerve damage, vision problems, and muscle weakness. British herbalist David L. Hoffmann, Ph.D. author of *The Herbal Handbook*, recommends EPO for MS.

PMS. Discomforts such as irritability, bloating, breast soreness, and depression occur before and during menstruation in many women. Clinical studies show that the GLA found in evening primrose oil contains essential fatty acids that seem to alleviate symptoms. A good friend of mine, Steven Morris, N.D., a naturopathic physician who practices near Seattle, Washington, prescribes evening primrose for PMS to good effect.

Raynaud's disease. Raynaud's disease is a condition that causes a loss of blood flow to the fingers, toes, nose, or ears. The affected areas turn white from the lack of circulation, then blue and cold, and finally numb. When the attack subsides, the affected parts may turn red and may throb, tingle, or swell. Research on GLA suggests that it can help relieve these symptoms. In one study, researchers massaged EPO into the fingers of people with the disease, and about half improved. I can't give EPO all the credit, though. I suspect that the massage helped to stimulate circulation, too.

Rheumatoid arthritis. Patients with this condition complain of chronic inflammation, pain, and tightness in the muscles or joints. When given evening primrose oil in one clinical trial, patients showed significant improvement and experienced less pain and stiffness in the morning. If I had arthritis, I'd take EPO capsules and apply the evening primrose oil topically, too. I wouldn't hesitate to take it daily, either, since there's not much to fear from a food "farmaceutical" like this.

How to Take It and How Much

You can take evening primrose in two forms: as seeds, or preferably, as standardized EPO supplements. Both contain GLA.

Seeds. If you use the seeds of the evening primrose, grind them first with a mortar and pestle, which I do when making my cornbread. I suspect that unmashed seeds pass straight through the digestive system undigested, which means you may eliminate—quite literally— the health benefits.

In the autumn, I'll often pass a patch of evening primroses on one of my nature walks through my Green Farmacy Garden. Since I don't have my mortar and pestle handy, I'll just shake the seeds from the plant into my palm and chew the unmashed seeds for a quick GLA fix, using my molars as mortars and pestles.

Supplements. For most people, I recommend taking standardized evening primrose oil preparations with specified levels of GLA. You have to eat an awful lot of seeds to get the equivalent of a standardized supplement, and buying the herb in capsules, or in bottle form as an extract, at your health food store is a far more practical alternative. Suggested dosages are usually two 1,300-milligram capsules per day or up to four to eight grams of evening primrose oil daily.

Useful Combinations

Taking evening primrose in conjunction with other herbs and foods can boost its healthful effects.

Borage and black currant oils. Borage and black currant, like evening primose, are rich in GLA and effective when taken in combination. While neither has been researched as thoroughly as evening primrose, studies suggest both may be effective in treating a variety of health complaints. In one study done at the University of California, San Francisco, borage oil lowered blood pressure in rats with hypertension. One caution: Unlike evening primrose oil, borage, the herb, is not safe for long-term use and should not be taken by pregnant or lactating women. The borage plant contains pyrrolizidine alkaloids.

Pumpkin or sunflower seeds. Like evening primrose seeds, these contain tryptophan, which boosts serotonin levels in the brain and acts as an herbal mood enhancer. Try eating all three types together as a kind of happy trail mix. Since many people tend to eat more when they're feeling blue, it's good to know that nibbling on these seeds can also curb the appetite. It's a chain reaction: Tryptophan raises your serotonin levels, and they turn around and tell your satiety centers you're not hungry anymore.

Saw palmetto. If you—like me—are concerned about prostate

health, take saw palmetto before you go with EPO. Saw palmetto has earned a rightful place in Duke's Dozen because it shows remarkable promise for keeping the prostate in good working order. (For more information on saw palmetto, see chapter 14.)

St. John's wort is another weapon in my herbal arsenal, covered in detail in chapter 13. Both St. John's wort and evening primrose calm skin irritations. To treat dermatitis, insect bites, or scabies (an itch caused by parasites under the skin), steep flowering shoots of St. John's wort for a few days in enough EPO to cover them, then dab the infused oil onto affected areas. If you don't have access to the fresh herb, you can use a tincture of St. John's wort.

The same herbal mixture may also provide relief for rheumatoid arthritis. Try smoothing it onto achy joints once a day.

FROM MY SCIENCE NOTEBOOK

Evening primrose is good for you in three ways.

First, its oil (EPO) is rich in gamma-linolenic acid (GLA), a fatty acid essential to human health. GLAs help make prostaglandins, compounds that perform such important bodily tasks as regulating brain function, blood flow, gastrointestinal activity, fluid balance, and fat decomposition. You'd have to search far and wide to find a better GLA source, as there are only a few other food sources that contain large quantities: borage, black currant, hemp seed oil, and mother's milk.

Second, evening primrose leaves are our best source of the bioflavonoid quercetin. Bioflavonoids are not produced by the human body but are found in many leaves, bark, seeds, and flowers, and they're important to good health. They protect blood vessels, aid in circulation, stimulate bile production, and lower cholesterol levels.

While evening primrose leaves are a good place to get your quercetin, they're not particularly tasty. If it's quercetin you're after, you might try mixing the young, tender, evening primrose leaves with onion, the second best source of quercetin, to make it more palatable. Better, perhaps, is a standardized supplement.

The third major active ingredient in evening primrose is tryptophan, an amino acid. The evening primrose seed (though not the oil) is one of the better sources of tryptophan. Your body converts some of it into serotonin, a brain chemical, which acts as a natural mood enhancer and antidepressant.

Stinging nettle. Along with evening primrose, stinging nettle is rich in quercetin, a bioflavonoid important to good health. Noted author Andy Weil, M.D., says he watched a hay-fever-suffering naturopathic experimenter swallow capsules of freeze-dried stinging nettle at an alternative medicines lecture at Columbia University in New York City. Her hay fever symptoms dried up in no time. People plagued by seasonal pollen allergies have learned that stinging nettle lets them to do away with antihistamines, drugs with significant toxicity and, often, undesirable side effects. Its efficacy in treating hay fever symptoms has been confirmed in one controlled clinical trial.

Friends who visit my nettle patch every spring take the herb and eat the greens as a food farmaceutical approach to hay fever. I also recommend my Sniffler's Soup, made by adding a handful of evening primrose leaves, two handfuls of stinging nettle, and one large diced onion to a favorite soup recipe.

Caution: Contraindications, Interactions, and Side Effects

Research on evening primrose looks clean. Like most food farmaceuticals, it's generally safe and causes far fewer side effects than most of its pharmaceutical alternatives. Still, keep an eye out for the following.

Headaches. Some scientific findings have shown that headaches and even nausea can occur in some people who take EPO. I heard one report from a friend who said she got migraines if she took large dosages of evening primrose seed for her PMS. She's not sure, I'm not sure, and the jury's still out until definitive studies are done.

Pharmaceutical alert. Schizophrenic patients on phenothiazines (Thorazine) may experience mild breathing difficulties or even increased risk of epilepsy, according to some research studies on such patients who took EPO.

Pregnancy and lactation. EPO is generally given the go-ahead for breastfeeding mothers, since GLA is found in breast milk. However, it's probably smart to stay on the safe side if you are pregnant or lactating. Consult your physician.

chapter seven

Garlic

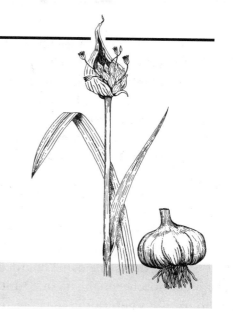

LATIN NAME: *Allium sativum*
FAMILY NAME: Alliaceae

TO SAY "GARLIC IS THE GREATEST" is no herbal hyperbole. This breathtaking bulb is one of the most versatile herbs around. It contains healthful chemicals and compounds galore, and it can be used to treat a remarkable variety of conditions and complaints. So it is with great confidence that I take some garlic almost every day and, coincidentally, why garlic is among America's best-selling herbs.

Garlic is best used for lowering blood pressure and lowering cholesterol, but since I am blessed with good ratings for both, I use garlic in the way that I use echinacea, as a booster for the immune system.

I also think garlic, like milk thistle, can protect the liver. In fact, I'm thinking of seeking a trademark for a better beer nut: a garlic coated milk thistle seed. Garlic can protect the liver from assorted toxins, including alcohol, and even heavy metals and pharmaceuticals like acetaminophen.

Both garlic and onion have also been proven to increase the body's defense mechanisms against bacteria and viruses. I've always believed that if you eat enough garlic, your body is better prepared to combat germs—and people, including people with colds, will stay away from you.

Although I've retired from my job as an ethnobotanist for the

U.S. Department of Agriculture, I feel my real work has just begun, and I still do a lot of traveling in the interest of herbal medicine. In the course of these long, stressful trips, I'll meet hundreds of people, some most likely suffering from a cold or flu, so this is when I take echinacea and garlic most conscientiously (although I take my garlic capsules *after* social functions are behind me).

Here's just one account of how I believe it helps. One recent spring day, I left my beautiful Green Farmacy Garden in Maryland and went west to Ohio State University, where I gave a lecture on herbal medicine to a house full of students. From Ohio, I headed to Seattle, where I presented a lecture sponsored by Nature's Herbs, at a regional meeting of the National Nutritional Foods Association.

Later that same day, I boarded a red-eye flight to Miami, where I caught another night flight to Lima, Peru, where I had a full three hours sleep before the final leg to the ReNuPeRu Garden in Amazonian Peru. It's a display garden where eco-tourists can visit and learn about 200 local medicinal plants growing there. It was constructed by my friend and shaman, Antonio Montero Pisco, and funded by me.

The garden, associated with the Amazon Center for Environmental Education and Research, is a wonderful place, just off a tributary of the Amazon and 2,300 miles upstream from the Atlantic Ocean. But when I arrived, the river's waters were higher than I had ever seen them, fully capable of flooding out village cesspools and country toilets.

My herbal immunostimulants and antiseptics (echinacea and garlic) apparently protected me, while three of the eco-tourists attending my one-week medicinal plant workshop suffered bouts of dehydration or gastrointestinal infection.

After more than two weeks away, I finally returned home. And thanks to a strong immune system and a good herbal regimen, I was in good health. I was happy to see the garlic coming up strong in my Green Farmacy Garden, where I grow it in a full one-quarter of the garden's 80 plots.

Garlic has an exceptionally long history as a medicinal plant, and for good reason. Here is my list for garlic: allergy, angina, asthma, bronchitis, burns and sunburn, cancer, cancer prevention, colds and flu, dermatitis, diabetes, earache, fungal infections, heart disease, herpes and cold sores, high blood pressure, HIV, leukemia and lymphoma, mastalgia (breast pain), sinusitis, ulcers, vaginitis, and yeast infections.

What Garlic Is and What It Can Do

Garlic is hardy and very easy to grow. Plants are tall and slim, and their leaves are long, flat, narrow, and graceful as they arise from the center of an underground cluster of cloves. These clusters are sometimes called heads of garlic, and they are encased in thin papery skins that can be white, gray, or mottled purple or rose. Mature plants can grow to be about four feet high, and their underground heads can be as large as an adult's fist.

Garlic is traditionally planted in the fall by burying individual cloves two to three inches deep. When harvested next summer, each clove will have multiplied itself to form a whole head.

With its strong flavor and pungent odor, garlic should be cut or crushed very finely and used in moderation for most purposes. If fried in oil that is too hot, garlic develops an acrid flavor. Garlic cloves are used fresh, dried, or powdered as a seasoning, rather than as a vegetable, although the tender, green parts of young garlic are widely eaten in China.

There are two main forms of the culinary garlic plant. One, sometimes called serpent or rocambole garlic, produces a curved, snakelike stalk topped by a round globe of little flowers. The other type, the kind most widely grown commercially, does not produce this flower stalk. After thousands of years, taxonomists are still debating whether each constitutes a separate species or whether they are variations of the same species.

A Worldwide Wonder

Garlic's vegetative homeland is Central Asia, but long ago its popularity spread to all parts of Europe, Asia, and North Africa,

(continued on page 112)

Garlic is older than recorded history. It was there when the Egyptians built the pyramids. Remnants of garlic were found in Tutankhamen's tomb (he died in 1352 B.C.). Herodotus, the "father of history," wrote that the laborers who built the pyramids were fed with radishes, onions, and garlic. And a manual from the time of the pyramids lists 22 medicines containing garlic.

When the children of Israel were lost, hungry, and wandering in the wilderness of Sinai, they had alliums on their mind. "We remember the fish, which we did eat in Egypt freely; the cucumbers, the melons, the leeks, the onions, and the garlic," they cried unto Moses in Numbers 11.

The first written references to garlic were found in Sumerian documents dating to the third millennium B.C., and this wonderful plant has been in print ever since. Every civilization from Africa to China seems to have valued its essence and left a record of its powers.

Hippocrates, the "father of medicine," prescribed eating garlic as treatment for uterine tumors. The Bower Manuscript, dating about A.D. 450 in India, recommended garlic for abdominal tumors and as an aphrodisiac. The Birch Bark Manuscript, found in Central Asia and written in Old Sanskrit, calls garlic a panacea, a remedy for all diseases. This is not far from the truth.

When I tabulate references to medicinal uses of garlic in folklore and old texts, I end up with a list of just about every condition you can think of. Sometimes I think it would be more challenging to find diseases that garlic was *not* used for.

Garlic Goes Native

When the first Paleolithic hunters followed their game across the Bering Strait out of Siberia and into the New World, they didn't find *Allium sativum* in North America. But these first immigrants brought with them genetic and mental recollections of many Russo/Sino/Tibetan foods and medicines they'd left behind. When they found allium plants here—there are about 150 native species—they recognized their value. By the time the Europeans arrived from the other direction, the first wave of immigrants had put about 30 species of allium to some good use.

In his monumental 1998 book, *Native American Ethnobotany*, Daniel E. Moerman, Ph.D., professor of anthropology at the University of Michigan, says that the primary medicinal uses of alliums were as cold remedies, as skin aids (often to prevent insect bites), and to ease breathing. My Amazonian shaman in Peru lists asthma, bronchitis, and tuberculosis first, not coincidentally.

The leading species, used widely by the Cherokee, Navaho, and Thompson Indians, was *Allium cernuum*, or "nodding onion," which today grows in southern Canada and throughout most of the United States. Research has tabulated a total of 78 uses, most as food, some as drug.

Among the first plants to sprout in the beginning of the year, alliums were a welcome spring tonic for many tribes. Their leaves contain vitamin C, which would have helped fight off colds and scurvy. Early European settlers quickly learned to appreciate the ramp (*Allium triccocum*), also called the wild leek, and springtime ramp food festivals survive throughout the Appalachians to this day.

All our wild alliums share many chemicals and biological activities with the more famous garlic. If I didn't have any cultivated garlic, I'd head outside and pick some wild garlic, *Allium vineale*. It's almost as rank as the ramp, but better than no garlic at all.

Garlic Repels Vampire Bats?

It was in Panama that I was inspired to start building my database of scientific information about the various substances in plants, because the natives there knew how to heal themselves with plants. I was very impressed and wanted to find the chemistry behind the folklore.

One of the most helpful things the Panamanians taught me was to rub garlic on my feet to keep the vampire bats from biting me while I was sleeping. I'm tall and my toes would sometimes protrude through the mosquito netting over my hammock. Sometimes I wonder what came first: garlic to repel vampire bats, or garlic to fight off Transylvanian terrors, but it works—I've had no trouble with either.

where garlic has been grown for food, spice, and medicine for thousands of years. (None of the synthetic drugs have been with us for 200 years, much less 2,000.)

I suspect that garlic was planted by the first farmers because its strong, complex flavor would have been a welcome addition to a bland, Neolithic diet. Early garlic lovers would soon have noted how the allium's antibiotic properties helped preserve food in a world without refrigerators. And if garlic helped preserve food, people soon figured out that it would help preserve them, too.

As civilization advanced (if that is the correct term), garlic was sure to be part of any herbal or medicinal record, from Egypt to China. By 1843, a popular family health guide published by George Friedrich Most in Germany gave garlic remedies for ear- and toothache ("put a fried garlic bulb on the upper arm; the skin will be reddened and thus the pain will be relieved through diversion"), for herpes rashes, for nerve deafness, for whooping cough, to eliminate worms, to prevent infectious diseases, for coughs and stomach trouble, for mad dog bites and snake bites, and to grow hair.

Today, third-world countries often rely on garlic as an expectorant in the treatment of tuberculosis, bronchial disorders, lupus, pulmonary gangrene, and inflammation of the trachea. Garlic is widely known as "Russian penicillin," because Russian physicians have long used it for respiratory disorders, giving children with whooping cough garlic ingredients via inhalation. Russians have also used garlic and onion preparations for flu, sore throats, and mouth sores.

DR. DUKE'S NOTES

Scientists in Bulgaria discovered that garlic given to afflicted lead mine workers considerably reduced their symptoms of poisoning.

It never ceases to amaze me that there is almost always a chemical or suite of chemicals in a plant that explains why it is used for its popular indications. Few herbs have more folklore attached to them than garlic, and few herbs have more phytochemicals that can give reason to the folklore.

All in all, the roster of garlic's biologically active compounds reads like a pharmacist's shelf—approximately 70 compounds have been identified so far. When I tabulated the effectiveness of garlic for

Compared to other plants, garlic contains an unusually high concentration of sulfur. Garlic is very rich in sulfur—containing more than three times the amount in apricots, broccoli, and onions, the foods with the next highest amounts.

Sulfur protects the garlic plant from invading fungi and bacteria as well as larger foes such as worms, nematodes, and other parasites. Above ground, garlic's strong flavor also protects it from animals that would eat its leaves. Even my voracious deer and groundhogs don't share my appetite for garlic.

Sulfur has long been recognized as an element that is useful in preventing or treating disease in the human body, too. It can be found in many modern medicines, including antibiotics, diuretics, and drugs that lower cholesterol and high blood pressure.

A whole clove of fresh garlic doesn't smell like sulfur until it's cut or crushed, and an amino acid called alliin is exposed to oxygen. This activates an enzyme called alliinase, which acts on alliin to produce garlic's active ingredient, allicin, a thiosulfinate. Allicin gradually breaks down into other sulfur compounds, depending on the conditions around it.

my database, I found clinical proof, or scientific experiments using humans, that garlic is indeed effective for heart problems, especially for lowering high blood pressure and cholesterol levels, and for thinning the blood, thereby lessening the likelihood of heart attack and stroke.

I also found other good, strong evidence for garlic's activity as an antibiotic and for the treatment of burns, cancer prevention, strengthening the immune system, and respiratory problems. And I found less conclusive, but very suggestive, evidence that garlic is helpful for arthritis, intestinal disorders and parasites, lead poisoning, tuberculosis, typhus, and senile dementia.

Garlic is readily accepted in Europe as a phytomedicinal, and of all the herbs in Duke's Dozen, I think garlic and ginkgo have made the biggest dent in the fortress of the physicians.

I would advise any serious student of garlic—and any medical doctor—to read *Garlic: The Science and Therapeutic Application of* Allium sativum *and Related Species*, edited by Heinrich P. Koch, Ph.D., and Larry D. Lawson, Ph.D. A real landmark in the study of this marvelous herb, this book cites more than 2,000 references to scientific studies of garlic's medicinal effects.

How Garlic Can Help

With all its biologically active compounds, a little clove of garlic is really nature's magic silver-skinned bullet. Here are some of its best-known, best-substantiated applications:

Altitude sickness. Garlic's antiaggregant properties might help it alleviate the symptoms of altitude sickness, according to U.S. Navy researchers at Bethesda. I spent my 65th birthday at Machu Picchu, Peru's famous Inca ruin, elevation 8,000 feet. Getting there, we gasped for air at the Cuzco airport, 12,000 feet above sea level.

When you go way above the clouds, your body has to adjust to a decreased oxygen supply. Fluids move from the blood to body tissues, and the result is thick blood and dehydration. So if you're planning to go mountain climbing, aggregate some of those antiaggregant veggies in a watery soup to prevent your blood from thickening up.

The Bethesda scientists also suggested that thymol, an ingredient in thyme (and many of the wild mints that grow around Machu Picchu) might help mountain sickness, too, so flavor your soup with this herb.

Arthritis. Arthritis is the name given to a number of different inflamed joint diseases from a number of different causes. Symptoms include swelling, pain, stiffness, and redness. Garlic contains more than a dozen anti-inflammatory compounds, several pain-relieving compounds, plus a couple compounds that reduce swelling.

As a gout sufferer (gout is one of the many kinds of arthritis), I was interested to read that the enzyme xanthine oxidase from the liver was inhibited by garlic. This enzyme is involved in chemical processes that lead to excess accumulations of uric acid, which cause terrible pain when deposited in joints. Cooked garlic was more effective at inhibiting this enzyme than fresh garlic juice, showing that something other than allicin is responsible, because allicin disappears after cooking.

Athlete's foot. Fungi love warm, damp, cozy places like the insides of shoes. I go barefoot whenever I can, and this goes a long way to prevent athlete's foot and its itchy, peeling, and cracked skin. But garlic can help, too. My first choice of treatment is a footbath once or twice a day made by putting several crushed cloves in a basin of warm water and a little rubbing alcohol.

Blood clots. Garlic contains compounds that are classified as antiaggregants, because they are very effective in keeping blood platelets from sticking together and clotting. This ability could be very helpful if your arteries are plugged with fatty deposits, because these can cause the blood to clot as it flows over the irregular surfaces of the deposits. Clotting, as well as those fat deposits, could block the artery and cause a heart attack.

When I researched the plants with the greatest variety of antiaggregant compounds, the result read like a spicy tofu salad. Garlic was the champion with nine different antiaggregants; tomato, dill, and

 A CASE IN POINT

Help for Athlete's Foot

At a recent symposium, I was approached by a man who said he was successfully controlling his toenail fungus with three different herbs, ranking them from most to least effective as walnut, garlic, and tea tree oil. Toenail fungus (onychomycosis) very frequently begins as athlete's foot, which then invades a toenail. Athlete's foot is fairly easy to control, but nail fungus is not easily controlled by anything. Most doctors are failing with the medical treatment of toenail fungus.

The man said his first line of defense was a footbath prepared with whole green walnut husks. For him, that was more successful than his independent trials of garlic footbaths and tea tree oil baths. All three of these are antifungals, but the one that's best for him may not be the one that's best for me, or the one that's best for you. Each of us is chemically different. So if I were to develop a problem with athlete's foot, I'd try all three, alone or maybe mixed together. I'd rather smell like tea tree than garlic.

Here's my garlic footbath remedy: Dice or crush 10 garlic cloves into a wash basin of warm water with a little lemon juice. Soak your feet for about 15 minutes, then dry them carefully. Don't do this before a social engagement, however—garlic's odiferous compounds can enter your body through the skin and exit through your mouth a little while later. You'll be able to taste them.

fennel each have seven; onion, hot pepper, and soybean have six; and celery, carrot, and parsley each have five. The more you add, the more you're protecting yourself from stroke, and the more likely you are to induce bleeding.

Blood pressure. Hypertension is often associated with increased risk for heart attack. In studies, garlic has been shown to lower blood pressure. It appears that something other than allicin is responsible. It may be adenosine, which enlarges blood vessels. Or it may be something that inhibits an enzyme that increases blood pressure. Or it may be something that increases the production of nitric oxide, which is associated with lower blood pressure. Whatever it is, garlic has it.

Cancer. Cancer is a group of diseases in which symptoms are due to unrestrained growth of cells, or malignant tumors, in body organs or tissues. Cancer begins when the genes controlling cell growth and multiplication are transformed by carcinogens. Once a cell is transformed into a tumor-forming type, it passes its change onto all offspring cells.

A number of recent epidemiological studies looked at cancer in relation to garlic consumption, and the results were very significant. In almost every study, eating garlic was linked to a reduced risk of cancer, especially in the gastrointestinal tract. Researchers suspect that garlic's allicin inhibits the formation of carcinogenic nitrosamines in the stomach.

> ## DR. DUKE'S NOTES
>
> *Surgeons in France and China have used the skin of garlic bulbs to help repair ruptured ear drums by covering the injured area with a layer of garlic cells to assist the healing process.*

In the very important five-year "Iowa Women's Health Study," published in 1994, researchers reported that garlic was the only food of 127 studied that showed a statistically significant association with a decreased risk of colon cancer. And all it took was one or more servings a week.

I have said in many lectures that if I were diagnosed with cancer, I'd probably go with herbal remedies instead of chemotherapy, and garlic would be one of the things that I would be taking. By taking garlic in combination with echinacea and turmeric for boosting the immune system, I'd have an herbal shotgun of phytochemicals, dozens of them, that would be attacking the cancer on different fronts.

Too often the chemotherapy weakens the patient more than it weakens the cancer, but when you go with the herbals, you're strengthening the patient and often weakening the cancer. That is the natural approach. Usually it's the sulfur-containing compounds that have anticancer activity, and garlic has more of these than any other herb I can think of.

Also, garlic contains the important trace element selenium at higher levels than found in most fruits and vegetables with the exception of cauliflower, spinach, mushrooms, and grains, where it is found at about the same levels, and asparagus, where it is three times as abundant. Selenium promotes antioxidant activity, which protects against cancer.

Garlic also contains substances that inhibit tumor activity. In experiments with mice, garlic extracts were shown to have an inhibitory effect on cancer cells.

Candidiasis. Infection by the fungus *Candida albicans* can upset the natural balance of microorganisms within the vagina, or less commonly on other areas of mucous membrane such as the mouth or on moist skin. The fungus occurs naturally in these moist areas and is usually kept under control by beneficial bacteria. Allowed to grow unchecked, however, the fungus infection can cause a thick, white discharge from the vagina with itching or painful urination.

I think garlic is one of the best herbs going for candidiasis. Study after study has shown the fungicidal effect of allicin on *Candida albicans.* In 1986, one research team found that garlic curtailed the fungus's ability to take up oxygen and inhibited its biosynthesis of protein and lipids. These effects show up in the blood soon after eating fresh garlic. Garlic also helps prevent an outbreak of candidiasis by boosting an impaired immune system to help fight it off.

Colds and flu. Sniffling, sneezing, coughing—we all know the symptoms of colds and flu. These viral infections cause inflammation and congestion of the nose and throat. As anyone who has ever had garlic breath knows, the herb's aromatic compounds are readily released from the lungs and respiratory tract, putting garlic's active ingredients right where they can be most effective against cold and flu viruses. Garlic is also an expectorant and will help your body clear up congestion.

Garlic works before the fact and after the fact—it is both germicidal and immune boosting. A Japanese study showed that garlic best protected mice from an influenza virus if they were fed a garlic extract for 15 days before infection. So I take it more as a preventive, but I would also take it if I were down with the flu. It certainly is going to work better than a synthetic antibiotic, which is wasted if you have a viral cold.

Heart health. Many people tell me how they have brought their cholesterol down and cleaned out their arteries with garlic, and it's true—what garlic can do for heart health is quite overwhelming. It contains at least five biologically active compounds that have been shown to help lower blood pressure, more than a dozen that lower cholesterol, and about a dozen that help reduce the risk of stroke and blood clots.

You've probably heard about "good," or high-density lipoprotein (HDL), cholesterol, and "bad," or low-density lipoprotein (LDL), cholesterol. Too much of the wrong kind of cholesterol can result in impaired blood supply due to blockage or narrowing of vessels by fat deposits. This is the major cause of heart disease in developed countries. Heart disease can manifest itself as angina, or chest pain usually associated with anxiety or effort, or a heart attack.

A high-fat diet, a sedentary lifestyle, and stress all contribute to heart disease. So can heart disease drugs—and each and every drug that lowers cholesterol may also offer some not-so-welcome side effects, such as liver or kidney problems, for example. What better way to safeguard your heart than by eating lots of low-fat salads and vegetables seasoned with lots of garlic? And since physical inactivity is a major risk factor, growing your own garlic in your garden would help, too. (While wearing a hat and sunscreen, of course.)

In a medical college study published in 1998, three scientists from Udaipur, India, found that daily doses of raw garlic extract significantly reduced total serum cholesterol and triglycerides, increased significantly HDL cholesterol, and produced other heart-healthy effects.

High cholesterol. Too much LDL can gum up your blood vessels with fat deposits, which harden into plaque. As vessels narrow, your body's blood supply is decreased. If your blood's platelets tend to aggregate, or your blood tends to clot, the blockage in the vessels increases, decreasing blood flow and increasing blood pressure. You're a candidate for heart disease. If your heart's blood supply is cut off, you could have a heart attack.

In study after study, garlic has been shown to be effective in lowering cholesterol levels. It is suspected that garlic re-

> ### DR. DUKE'S NOTES
> *The former Soviet Union once imported 500 tons of garlic during an influenza epidemic.*

duces cholesterol (serum lipids) by decreasing fat absorption. The evidence points to allicin or allicin-derived ingredients as the component of garlic that is responsible. The sulfur in garlic inactivates the sulfur in human gastric lipase, the enzyme involved in the absorption of fats. The Russians even have a brand-name garlic preparation for people with arteriosclerosis, or thickened, stiff artery walls.

Garlic got an unfair rap—and negative media attention—in 1998, when *The Journal of the American Medical Association (JAMA)* published an article to the effect that garlic does *not* lower cholesterol. The study had been based on how 25 people had taken a garlic product, Tegra, a pill containing concentrated garlic oil that is sold in Germany. After six weeks, the authors found no lowering of the subjects' cholesterol levels. The fault of this research was that Tegra does not contain the major cholesterol-lowering compounds of garlic. It's prepared from a steam-distilled oil of garlic, in which the allicin is converted into various oil-soluble compounds.

Dr. Lawson, co-author of the previously mentioned excellent book on garlic, wrote a rebuttal to this study that was subsequently published in *JAMA*. Dr. Lawson also found that Tegra passes through the body undigested. Since the subjects took Tegra, not garlic, it was not a study of garlic at all; it was a study of Tegra.

In their book, Drs. Koch and Lawson reviewed 40 clinical garlic studies and found that garlic can lower cholesterol by an average of 10 percent or more and can lower triglycerides, which also carry fat in the blood, by an average of 13 percent. They are almost all European studies, which don't tend to be quite as biased as our American studies. So I'll stick with my whole garlic, believing as I did before that a clove of garlic a day will keep the hypocholesterolemic hucksters away.

HIV infection. Acquired immune deficiency syndrome, or AIDS, is caused by the human immunodeficiency virus (HIV). This virus weakens the body's immune system, opening the door to many opportunistic infections and cancers. Complications from AIDS require treatment with antibiotics, and garlic is one of the best herbal antibiotics. If I had AIDS, I'd certainly be taking garlic every day.

Garlic helps combat many of the secondary infections, including pneumonia, candidiasis, and herpes. Garlic also acts as an immune stimulant. A 1988 study showed that when volunteers ate either raw garlic (with allicin present) or aged garlic extract (with allicin absent), their natural killer cell activity in the blood doubled. There's also some

 ## WHAT NEW RESEARCH TELLS US

Here's an update on what new research into garlic has revealed about possible new uses for this versatile herb:

HPS Syndrome. Medical doctors are at a loss when it comes to hepatopulmonary syndrome (HPS)—no therapy exists for this condition, marked by poor oxygenation of blood and shortness of breath. After an HPS patient was reported to have improved by eating garlic regularly, researchers at the University of Alabama at Birmingham set out to determine if they could repeat the results. They gave garlic powder capsules to 15 patients daily. After six months, almost half had improved.

Peptic ulcers. From China comes the first demonstration that garlic can kill *Helicobacter pylori*, the bacteria associated with peptic ulcers. Researchers at China Medical College in Taichung, Taiwan, found that sulfur-containing compounds in garlic inhibit an enzyme in the microorganism.

evidence that garlic compounds can kill HIV-1 infected cells directly.

Infections. As an antibiotic, garlic helps fight infection when the body is invaded by bacteria, a virus, or a fungus. In their book, Drs. Koch and Lawson list over 30 organisms that garlic has been shown to work against.

Garlic's antibiotic effect is mainly due to allicin and its sulfur content. Several studies show that allicin may attack enzymes inside bacteria's cell walls. It also seems to inhibit bacteria's RNA (ribonucleic acid) synthesis, which, in turn, would keep the bacteria from multiplying. What's more, garlic boosts an impaired immune system as well as prevents infection when the immune system is impaired. Together, your immune system *and* the garlic can attack the disease better.

> ## DR. DUKE'S NOTES
>
> *As an antioxidant, garlic inhibits the formation of free radicals, those trouble-causing, unbalanced molecular pieces or atoms that break up or bind with any molecules they come in contact with in the body. Garlic also strengthens radical scavengers and protects low-density lipoprotein against oxidation, or breakdown, by free radicals.*

I do think of garlic as the poor man's penicillin—but better, because penicillin is only one drug with one type of active ingredient, and garlic is many drugs. Garlic is the herbal shotgun containing at least 25 germ-killing compounds. You are not going to develop resistance to it as quickly as you might to a single antibiotic. When you try to fight a bug with a single magic bullet antibiotic, it rapidly develops resistance, but if you give that bug garlic, or garlic *and* an antibiotic, resistance will be less likely because the germ is being attacked on several fronts.

Garlic also synergistically enhances the action of synthetic antibiotics. *E. coli* bacteria is becoming harder and harder to control, and recently people have died or become seriously ill after eating foods contaminated by a new, stronger strain. In a recent study, researchers compared a garlic and water extract (made by crushing 500 grams of garlic cloves in 150 milliliters of water), pure allicin, and two antibiotics, ampicillin and kanamycin. The garlic extract and the pure allicin were significantly more effective in killing *E. coli* bacteria than the synthetic antibiotics.

ALL IN THE FAMILY: ONION

Garlic comes from a big family. The *Allium* genus contains at least 450 species. Most are wild, but garlic has some well-known cultivated cousins, including onions, leeks, shallots, and chives. I believe that many of the benefits that accrue to garlic will accrue to other alliums, at least those that have a similar odor—it's those beneficial sulfur compounds at work.

I used to love a hot dog topped with mustard and onions. Then one day, I found that I could eat a piece of bread topped with mustard and onions and hot sauce, and I'd enjoy it almost as much. Now I eat this concoction so often it even has a name—I call it a "hot doggone." If you've got to have junk food, the least you can do is to try to make it a little healthful.

I don't mean to say that onions are in any way junk food. They are high fiber, low calorie, and provide some vitamin C and folate, a nutrient essential to pregnant women. And after wheat, they are, with garlic, our second major dietary source of inulin.

Onions contain a lot more water (about 90 percent) than garlic (about 60 to 65 percent), but they have many of the same sulfur compounds that make garlic so valuable. I could plant onions in the same ailment beds here in the Green Farmacy Garden as I have the garlic, since I consider them generic substitutes.

What Onion Is and What It Can Do

Onion plants are similar to garlic plants—tall, skinny green leaves growing from the center of an underground bulb. Instead of multiple cloves, however, onions have fleshy, concentric layers encased in an outer skin that can be yellow, white, or red. Onions can be extra large—one seed company touts soccer ball–size onions—or extra small, like the kind you find pickled in little jars.

Onions are a very popular food eaten around the globe, both as a flavoring and as a vegetable. Whole onions may be served boiled, baked, creamed, or sliced. Young green onions, often called scallions, add spice to salads and stir-fries.

Onions hail from the same part of the world as garlic: Central Asia and the Near East. Today, onions are grown in many parts of North America—sweet onions like the Vidalia in the South and storage onions in the North.

Onion folklore calls it useful for angina, arteriosclerosis, asthma, bronchitis, coughs, dehydration, diabetes, digestion, the gallbladder, and high blood pressure and as a menstrual aid. Externally, onion has been applied to insect bites, bruises, boils, minor burns, warts, and wounds. A classic cold remedy is made by steeping raw onion slices overnight in honey.

As is the case for garlic, modern science is finally getting around to substantiating thousands of years of medicinal usefulness. And as can be expected with closely related plants, onions have many of the same health benefits.

Like garlic, onions contain alliin, which is broken down by enzymatic action into allicin and other therapeutic sulfur-containing compounds. Onions have only about a third as much sulfur as garlic, so in some cases, particularly heart health, garlic is considered the more effective herb by some people.

However, if you find it easier to eat three times as much onion as garlic (I enjoy onions more than garlic, myself), you'll get an equal amount of sulfur-containing compounds. (Some people who are allergic to garlic claim not to be allergic to onions.)

Where Onions Beat Garlic

Onions are clearly a better source of quercetin—48,100 ppm (parts per million) for onion bulbs compared to 200 ppm for garlic. Quercetin is a bioflavonoid. More than 50 activities have been ascribed to it, including inhibiting tumors, thinning the blood, lowering blood pressure, and relieving asthma and pain. In the herbal database I've compiled, quercetin comes up as the most effective compound for anti-inflammatory bowel disease.

In its pure form, quercetin is actually being sold now as an anti-allergy supplement for asthma and hay fever, but I don't recommend this. It may be completely harmless; it may not be. I prefer it in its natural context. That way you get all the synergy, "the symphony of nutrients working synergistically" that provides the great healing power of whole foods.

How Onions Can Help

Just like garlic, onions can help prevent heart disease by lowering cholesterol, lowering blood pressure, and helping to thin the blood. And like garlic,

(continued)

onions are useful for treating allergies, colds, diabetes, HIV infection, pneumonia, and yeast infections. But there are a few ailments onions are better for.

Asthma. Bronchial asthma is a chronic respiratory illness that now affects about 14 million Americans. Asthma is becoming a more serious problem, too—the number of people who die each year from complications of asthma attacks has increased over 30 percent since 1980.

Doctors can't explain this rise in asthma, but I believe that increased pollution, both outdoor and indoor, as well as fewer natural foods (and hence, less quercetin) in our national diet all play a part.

When asthma attacks, sensitive bronchial tubes constrict, making breathing difficult. The body also produces excess mucus, making it even harder to breathe. In one study, alcoholic extracts of onion (and garlic) were surprisingly active against chronic asthma, perhaps by inhibiting histamine (quercetin is a natural antihistamine) and/or by inhibiting enzymes that promote the production of irritants and other allergenic compounds.

Diabetes. In Asia, onions have long been a traditional remedy for people with diabetes. Recently, studies have shown that quercetin has helped with eye problems associated with diabetes, including cataracts and diabetic retinopathy, or damage to the back of the eye. Researchers suspect that quercetin inhibits an enzymatic process having to do with cataract formation.

How to Take It and How Much

Attempts to deodorize garlic can cause considerable changes in its composition, including removal of some of the main medicinal principles, since these are also responsible for the odor. People always ask me if deodorized garlic works as a medicinal. I always answer, "If the stinking rose don't stink it don't work. The fresher the garlic is right out of the soil, the better." That's my personal opinion, although I know it flies in the face of some of the research sponsored by the "odorless" garlic products.

Heating or cooking garlic can also change garlic's medicinal properties, because heating destroys the enzyme that creates allicin. However, since garlic is so biologically complex and active, there's

How to Take It and How Much

I eat onions almost every day, just like garlic. I add both onions and garlic to all my soups and most of my salads and veggie dishes. According to studies, half an onion is equal to one clove of garlic. But if you take the water out, onions are probably just as effective as garlic.

Like garlic, onions are best eaten raw if what you need is an antibiotic. However, if it's quercetin you're after, you're better off getting it from onion skins. I wouldn't eat those outer skins—they are pretty tough—but you can add them to soups and stews and fish them out before serving.

I think onions are so flavorful, they make everything else taste better, too. If I had asthma, I'd be eating nettle soup loaded with onion. Noted authority Dr. Andrew Weil, a well-known physician, thinks nettles are the best plant remedy for asthma.

Evening primrose leaves are not very tasty, but they are our best source of quercetin. So I mix them with onion, the second-best source of quercetin, to make evening primrose more palatable. I call this combination the "quercefix" and like to mix it with a combination of "crucifers" (broccoli, cauliflower, kale, mustard, turnips, watercress), with their pungent, anti-cancer isothiocyanates, as a dietary panacea.

more going on inside a clove than the sulfur compounds. Those previously mentioned epidemiological studies that associated a decreased cancer risk with garlic consumption didn't differentiate between cooked garlic and raw garlic. And since garlic is mainly eaten cooked, I think allicin is just the tip of the iceberg. So if it's a choice between cooked garlic or no garlic, I say go ahead and eat it cooked.

At the very least, I'd recommend eating at least one average clove, or about 4 grams, of fresh garlic per day to maintain health. If you are fighting something off, I'd suggest taking three to five cloves a day as a therapeutic dose. (Just to be clear about this, a clove is *one little individual piece* of garlic; the garlic *head* is a cluster of cloves.)

If you prefer the taste of cooked garlic, I'd estimate that you'd have to eat about four cloves to equal the effect of one fresh one. One average clove is also the equivalent of approximately 5,000 micrograms of allicin per day, or 400 milligrams of standardized garlic extract per day.

In a 1993 comparison of commercial garlic products, Dr. Lawson reported that garlic powder tablets contained about two-thirds as much allicin as fresh garlic. My biased reading of his summary is that fresh garlic is the best source of allicin and total sulfur compounds and that a well-made, standardized garlic powder pill is almost as good.

Almost every day when I'm at home I'll make a vegetable soup with whatever ingredients are on hand. Besides pretty well taking care of half my veggie quota for the day, the soups always have one to five cloves of garlic and up to half an onion in them. I throw in the garlic cloves whole with their skins still on, because these outer coverings probably contain more of the beneficial bioflavonoid quercetin than the internal part of the clove. (Bioflavonoids are substances found in plants that can have anti-allergy, anti-inflammatory, and antiviral activity.) My secretary, Judi, and I always fight to see who gets to eat the garlic.

Instead of soup, sometimes I'll make a fresh veggie juice by blending two cloves of garlic with two to four carrots and four stalks of celery. Because I suffer from gout, I take either celery seed or celery each day, and this is an easy way to kill two birds with one stone. The juice is amazingly calm tasting and mild smelling from what you would expect of something made with fresh garlic. Mrs. Duke says she doesn't

DR. DUKE'S RECIPES

Daily Beans

Legumes have so many beneficial effects that I try to eat them every day. One of my favorite ways is in a bean soup. My bean soups have a cup of dry beans soaked overnight. (Everyone else throws the soaking water away the next day, but not me—even though that water is flatugenic, some of those flatus-inducing compounds might prevent cancer.) Then I cook the beans with diced carrots (a folk remedy for reducing flatus), adding two to five whole cloves of garlic, one-half to one onion, some curry powder for its turmeric, a little hot sauce (also a cancer preventer), and black pepper (piperine in black pepper often synergizes or increases the effect of other "foodiceuticals"). A little olive oil is optional, but I like to top my bean soup with raw chopped onions and cilantro.

smell garlic on my breath this way as much as she notices it when I take garlic capsules, even the so-called "odor-free" kind.

Useful Combinations

Evolution favors synergy among compounds that protect the plant from its natural enemies. Different herbs can work together, too.

Echinacea. Because both echinacea and garlic are immunity boosters, I assume I'll benefit a little more if they both are part of my daily regimen than if I'm taking only one. (For more information about how echinacea helps to bolster your immune system and ward off colds and flu, see chapter 5.)

Hawthorn. Commercial preparations of garlic for lowering blood pressure sometimes also contain hawthorn, an herb that can dilate blood vessels and improve circulation. I advise heart-wary friends to eat the two as foods. (For more information on hawthorn, see chapter 9.)

Legumes. Genistein, the component that gives soy its lofty reputation, contains a phytochemical also found in other legumes. It has been found to retard cancer growth in test tubes—possibly by inhibiting the new blood vessel growth on which tumors depend.

I'd rather my daughter eat a bowl of beans than take a drug for the prevention or treatment of breast cancer. Since human beings co-evolved with plants, our genes know genistein, but they only met cancer-fighters such as raloxifene 4 years ago and tamoxiphen about 25 years ago.

So, because garlic and onion are mandatory ingredients when I cook legumes, and because I'm a cancer candidate (both my father and two of his brothers died of colon cancer at age 65), I try to eat one or two servings of beans each day. Some American beans may not have as much genistein as the soybean, but I eat more of them and that compensates for that.

Turmeric, onion, and burdock. If I had cancer, I'd be eating a lot of garlic, turmeric, onion, and burdock. When the body is out of whack, it can reach into the potpourri and find the things that it needs. The body has thousands of homeostatic equations going on, and these equations know what to grab from what you offer and to exclude the things you don't need.

Caution: Contraindications, Interactions, and Side Effects

Garlic is on the Food and Drug Administration's GRAS list, a list of food additives that are "generally recognized as safe" by a consensus of scientific opinion. A clove a day is well within the safe limit.

Allergy alert. I must caution, however, that there are people who are allergic to garlic. Eating a normal amount may cause gastrointestinal distress. Or rubbing a cut clove on their skin might burn more than expected.

Stomach irritation. Eating garlic on an empty stomach may irritate *anyone's* mucous membrane and result in heartburn and other pains. It's also possible to eat too much garlic. More than five cloves a day may cause flatulence and heartburn. And extremely high doses, the equivalent of eating 500 cloves of raw garlic a day, can damage the liver.

Prescription medication alert. While garlic's blood thinning effects can be beneficial to some, people who are already taking synthetic blood thinners may overthin their blood with garlic. One garlic lover's blood took twice as long to clot when she was on garlic than when she wasn't. It's important to talk to your doctor about *any* herbs you take, especially if you are taking prescribed medication.

Take care when eating garlic. How you eat your garlic can have an effect, too. When a 65-year-old man swallowed a whole garlic clove, the result was an intestinal occlusion, and he was saved only by emergency surgery, according to Koch and Lawson. I certainly do not recommend swallowing garlic cloves whole.

Botulism warning. Finally, I must mention that improper handling of garlic may result in botulism poisoning. It's tempting to put garlic into a bottle of olive oil to flavor the oil for salads, but this could be deadly. A number of cases of botulism were traced to unrefrigerated sandwich spreads made with chopped garlic, water, and oil. Steeping garlic cloves in vinegar is safe, however.

chapter eight

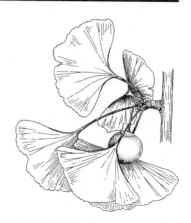

Ginkgo

LATIN NAME: *Ginkgo biloba*
FAMILY NAME: Ginkgoaceae

I STARTED TAKING GINKGO only in the last year, after I read a study in *The Journal of the American Medical Association* that acknowledged that ginkgo might help slow the effects of old age on the brain, which they called senile dementia.

Senile dementia is a blanket term for getting addled in your old age, and it includes Alzheimer's disease. Both my mother and her mother were sharp into their late nineties, but who knows what genes I may have inherited from my father's side—he died at age 65, too young for me to find out how he would have aged. I don't know nearly as much about my father's side of the family as my mother's. They were all much shorter lived.

So I'm taking ginkgo as a preventive, not for anything chronic. One doesn't notice any changes when one prevents something, and so far, I'd say the ginkgo is doing the job.

One of the ways it works is by improving circulation, both in the brain and in the body's extremities. Old folks often have poor circulation in their hands and feet, and ginkgo has been shown to help both of those. It also improves circulation in the sexual organs, another body extremity. Some California studies have also attributed an aphrodisiac effect to ginkgo extract.

My own personal experiments didn't indicate that, but I was taking whole, fresh ginkgo leaves, and I wouldn't recommend them to anybody. They might cause a poison ivy–like rash in particularly sensitive people.

What Ginkgo Is and What It Can Do

The ginkgo tree is a living fossil. The species that lines city sidewalks today is virtually the same tree that shaded dinosaurs in the Jurassic period. *Ginkgo biloba* is so old that it once grew widely throughout the northern hemisphere at a time when lands bordering the Arctic Ocean were warm and balmy.

All (Alone) in the Family

In the remote past, there were many species of ginkgo, but now *Ginkgo biloba* is an only child. It has the unique distinction of being the only species in the only genus in the only family in a single order of trees that have swimming sperm—that is, sperm that swim to the egg in the fertilization process. (It's true that some primitive plants have swimming sperm. Plants are a lot more like us than we think.)

Young ginkgoes have a narrow pyramid shape, but mature ginkgo trees can be wide and rounded and can reach more than 100 feet tall. Usually only male trees are planted, because the fruit of female trees smells like rancid butter due to the presence of butyric acid.

Ginkgo leaves are two to three inches across, stiff, flat, and fan-shaped, with a central indentation. (The species name, *biloba* is Latin for "bi-lobed.") Another name for the ginkgo is maidenhair tree, because its leaves are somewhat suggestive of the leaves of the maidenhair fern, which also have the same, unusual Y-shaped leaf veins.

DR. DUKE'S NOTES

Sales of ginkgo extract in Europe have totaled as much as $500 million per year.

The climate changes of the Ice Age put an end to the ginkgo in Europe. Elsewhere, it is said to have been all but extinct except for the trees carefully tended around monasteries and temples in China and Japan.

Ginkgoes can live for more than 1,000 years and have a vener-
ated role in traditional Asian medicine. Almost 5,000 years ago, the
Chinese used ginkgo leaves to prevent memory loss due to age, according to Georges Halpern, M.D., Ph.D., in his book *Ginkgo, A
Practical Guide*. The Chinese also burned the leaves and inhaled the
smoke to treat respiratory ailments, but mostly they valued ginkgo's
seeds and fruit.

WHAT NEW RESEARCH TELLS US

Recent research and experience has shown us some exciting new possibilities for ginkgo:

Sickle cell anemia. Medical herbalist Alan Keith Tillotson and his wife,
Naixin Hu Tillotson, a Chinese medicine specialist, run the Chrysalis Natural Medicine Clinic in Wilmington, Delaware. They report four startling
successes with sickle cell anemia, an inherited blood disease for which
medical doctors have no cure. Their herbal formula includes ginkgo plus
prickly ash bark (*Zanthoxylum*).

Radiation sickness. After the nuclear accident in 1986 at Chernobyl in
the Ukraine, emergency crews came from all parts of the former Soviet
Union to shut down the damaged reactor. Afterward, most of these workers
had increased levels of free radicals in their blood, putting them at risk for
chromosome damage and cancer. A French study published in 1995 reported that when these workers took 40 milligrams of ginkgo extract three
times a day for eight weeks, their levels of free radicals had fallen to normal
and were even maintained for seven months without further treatment.

Cellulite. Recently, ginkgo extracts have been showing up in cellulite
remedies, thanks to their ability to reduce swelling and improve blood flow
through the capillaries. Yes, those unique ginkgo constituents that can help
a body function better can make it look better, too. One research study
found that ginkgo was just as effective at reducing swelling due to irritation as indomethacin, a generic nonsteroidal anti-inflammatory drug.

Other researchers showed that ginkgo's ability to increase blood flow in
the capillaries, thus increasing skin temperature, can improve the condition and appearance of weak, sagging skin due to aging, as well as the appearance of dimpled skin, or cellulite.

Keeping Mentally Fit

In the West, we've only started to seriously look at ginkgo in the past few decades, and our modern applications of ginkgo are often different from what the Chinese used it for. Most of the recent medical research has been done in Germany on highly concentrated ginkgo leaf extracts used to improve peripheral circulation and to thin the blood.

There's good European research showing that by helping to improve blood flow to the brain, ginkgo counteracts some consequences of aging. Some studies, including one that I read in a 1997 *JAMA*, suggest that ginkgo helps people with Alzheimer's disease and other forms of dementia. Patients seem to become more alert and sociable, think more clearly, feel better, and remember more.

In Europe, a concentrated extract of the leaves is the top-selling pharmaceutical and is taken regularly by many older people to help keep themselves mentally fit.

How Ginkgo Can Help

Ginkgo's beneficial effects can be broken down into three categories: It protects cell health, cleans up free radicals, and keeps blood vessels strong. These actions can be very useful in treating and preventing a number of diseases and conditions. Here are a few of ginkgo's most notably proven applications.

Aging (memory problems, poor circulation, depression, etc.). Aging is a natural part of life—in time, our bodies slow down and weaken, and so do our brains. However, many hazards of old age—including poor memory, confusion, depression, and minor physical complaints such as dizziness—are not inevitable and can be slowed, some even reversed. Just as exercise, a balanced diet rich in phytochemicals, and sensible habits can keep our bodies in good condition for as long as we inhabit them, such practices can keep our brains going strong, too.

Ginkgo is a premier example of a substance that can keep your brain sharp by stimulating blood flow and brain function. Ginkgo

Ginkgo contains two main categories of active components—flavonoids and terpenes.

Flavonoids can be very beneficial, because they are antioxidants that can neutralize free radicals and protect the body from their ravages. Free radicals are those trouble-causing, unbalanced molecular pieces or atoms that break up or bind with any molecules they come in contact with wherever they are in the body.

Free radicals are believed to be involved with inflammation, degenerative diseases such as cancer and heart and circulatory diseases, and the aging process. Moreover, cerebral oxidative damage by free radicals can impair memory.

Flavonoids also maintain arachidonic acid, an unsaturated fatty acid that is needed for healthy cells. In addition, flavonoids are the components of ginkgo that improve circulation, reduce the tendency of blood platelets to stick together, protect blood vessels, and strengthen capillary walls.

Ginkgo's terpenes are in the form of substances called bilobalides and ginkolides, rare substances that occur only in ginkgo. Like ginkgo's flavonoids, many of its terpenes are antioxidants, too. But terpenes also improve circulation and metabolism, protect the body against unwanted blood clots, and protect nerve cells from damage. The terpenes have been credited with improving memory and mental function, and can help during recovery from a stroke.

As summarized by Commission E, Germany's government-appointed panel of physicians, pharmacologists, and other experts who review herbal medicines for safety and effectiveness, ginkgo:

➤ Increases the body's tolerance to lack of oxygen, especially in brain tissue
➤ Inhibits swelling (edema) in the brain caused by trauma or toxins
➤ Reduces swelling and lesions in the retina
➤ Inhibits age-related decline of choline receptors and promotes choline uptake in the brain
➤ Improves memory and learning capacity
➤ Helps with balance
➤ Improves blood flow, especially in the capillaries
➤ Scavenges free radicals
➤ Inhibits the platelet activating factor, a mediator of chemical processes within the body, including platelet aggregation, blood clotting, and allergic reactions
➤ Protects the nerves

contains unique terpene lactones, substances that help increase circulation to the brain and other parts of the body. These substances can also help protect nerve cells.

Remember that cerebral circulation is reduced in older people, and that's where ginkgo also helps by allowing more blood, and therefore more oxygen and glucose (blood sugar), to reach the brain's cells.

Hundreds of European studies have confirmed the use of standardized ginkgo leaf extract for a wide variety of conditions associated with aging, including memory loss and poor circulation. At the University of Vienna, researchers tested the effects of ginkgo on 48 patients between 51 and 79 years old with age-associated memory impairment. Results, published in Germany, showed that after 57 days, those taking the ginkgo extract experienced a slight improvement.

Another common condition of aging is depression. One European study recruited 40 depressed elderly people with cerebral blood flow problems who had not improved by taking pharmaceutical antidepres-

 HERB LORE AND MORE

The Chinese revere three legendary emperors who gave them wisdom and knowledge 5,000 years ago. One, the Emperor Shen Nung, is considered to be the first Chinese herbalist and is author of an ancient medical text, *Pen T'sao Ching*. In it, ginkgo leaves are said to help the elderly preserve their memory, and to aid breathing problems.

Chinese herbalists used ginkgo seeds to counteract diseases such as asthma or chronic diarrhea. Even today, roasted ginkgo seeds are served at celebrations in Japan and China because they are thought to aid digestion and prevent drunkenness. The seeds do actually contain two compounds shown to speed up the metabolism of alcohol, which has inspired my couplet:

They say that you won't get real stinko
If you nibble the nuts of the ginkgo.

sants. After taking 80 milligrams of ginkgo extract three times a day, both their depression and mental faculties had improved significantly.

Allergies. Dust, pollen, foods, pets, and plants—allergies to certain substances can be irritating (sneezing and itchy eyes) or life threatening (anaphylactic shock). When the body is exposed to allergens, cells release histamine. This causes blood vessels to swell, fluids to leak into tissues, and muscles to spasm. As a result, we experience the unpleasant symptoms associated with allergies, such as red, itchy, or swollen skin, sneezing and congested airways, or red, irritated eyes.

Ginkgo extract contains several unique compounds to counteract allergies, including seven antihistamines and a dozen anti-inflammatories.

Another substance released in an allergic reaction is called the platelet activating factor (PAF), which causes spasms of the bronchial muscles. Ginkgo's ginkgolides counteract PAF, thus lessening allergic reactions.

Altitude sickness. Ginkgo can prevent headaches by helping the lungs and brain use oxygen more efficiently—important when you are 10,000 feet above sea level, where oxygen levels are low. Studies have shown that standardized extracts of ginkgo leaves increase the flexibility of blood vessels in the brain, which improves circulation.

Ginkgo also thins the blood, which tends to thicken at high altitudes. Oxygen-rich blood can help reduce the headaches, dizziness, and confusion that often accompany altitude sickness. Brigitte Mars, a member of the American Herbalists Guild who teaches at the Rocky Mountain School of Botanical Medicine, in Boulder, Colorado, suggests starting to take ginkgo capsules several days before a trip to high elevations; the usual dose is 120 milligrams per day.

Alzheimer's disease. Alzheimer's disease is the most common cause of something doctors generally refer to as senile dementia. Alzheimer's affects about 4 million Americans. About 10 percent of people over age 65 can expect to suffer from the mental deterioration associated with the disease. If you live beyond age 85, your chances are one in two that you'll be diagnosed with Alzheimer's.

The symptoms of Alzheimer's are due to progressive deterioration of brain cells and vary from person to person. Most often, memory loss is the first sign, followed by disorientation and an inability to concentrate, calculate, or communicate. Final stages include hallucinations, delusions, and loss of control.

Ginkgo's potential for lessening the effects of Alzheimer's disease is found in its antioxidant properties. Ginkgo has a number of substances that work together to scavenge for free radicals, which are linked to the excessive oxidation and cell damage associated with Alzheimer's disease.

DR. DUKE'S NOTES

In 1999, the American Chemical Society awarded its Cope Award to E. J. Corey for the first synthesis of ginkgolides. It's interesting to see the great emphasis chemists put on trying to synthesize what nature has been kind enough to provide for free, in abundance, and in synergy with many more active compounds.

Ginkgo has recently been approved in Germany for the treatment of dementia, and there are many European studies to support this. In such studies, ginkgo extract improved the attention and memory of patients with senile or presenile dementia of the Alzheimer's type.

In 1998, Barry S. Oken, M.D., reviewed 50 studies in which Alzheimer's patients took ginkgo, and he concluded that ginkgo is almost as good at improving cognitive functions like alertness, attention, and memory as the synthetics approved by the U.S. Food and Drug Administration (FDA).

Asthma. Bronchial asthma is a chronic respiratory illness. When asthma attacks, sensitive bronchial tubes constrict, making breathing difficult. The body also produces excess mucus, making it even harder to breathe. Ginkgo contains numerous natural antihistamine compounds, which can help block the effects of histamine, a chemical that is released during an allergic reaction.

Another substance released is the platelet activating factor, a protein in the blood that plays a role in triggering bronchospasms. Ginkgo contains compounds called ginkgolides that inhibit PAF. Herbalists think ginkgo could be helpful by improving some types of allergies linked to asthma. Ginkgo's ginkgolides are antiallergens that can protect the bronchial tubes from substances that set off asthma attacks.

Broken capillaries and varicose veins. Ginkgo contains good quantities of rutin and other substances that strengthen capillaries. My taking bilberry, ginkgo, and horse chestnut may be a triple whammy for those leaky capillaries. As a highly effective treatment for various blood vessel disorders, ginkgo can have a toniclike effect to keep varicose veins from getting worse.

Eczema. People with eczema often have allergies that sensitize overreactive skin, causing redness and itching. Ginkgo can work inside the body to help decrease hypersensitivity to allergens. And when reactions are reduced, you get symptom relief.

Impotence. Impotence, or erectile dysfunction, is the inability to achieve or maintain an erection for sexual penetration or sexual satisfaction. Most men have experienced it at least once by the time they are age 40.

Erections are the result of a complex combination of brain stimuli, blood vessel and nerve function, and hormonal actions. Anything that interferes with any of these factors can cause impotence. Psychological factors such as stress, or side effects from drugs, can be the culprit. (My unfortunate first time was at age 16: forest near Grandfather Mountain, North Carolina; no blanket, probable rattlesnakes. In this case, laughter by my partner, later to become my first wife, cured all.) However, if poor geriatric circulation contributes to a case of impotence, you could try ginkgo as a circulatory stimulant to boost the blood flow to the penis.

Physicians have obtained very good results by prescribing 60 to 240 milligrams daily of a standardized ginkgo extract. In one nine-month study, 78 percent of men with impotence due to atherosclerotic clogging of the penile artery reported significant improvement without side effects. In another six-month study, half of the men being treated with ginkgo regained their erections.

Intermittent claudication (lameness). Intermittent claudication is another name for the lameness or limping that accompanies or follows short walks in the aging. The usual cause is a blockage or narrowing of arteries in the legs due to atherosclerosis, the clogging up of arteries associated with high cholesterol and thickened blood. Patients of intermittent claudication find that they have to stop walking after a set distance because of pain in the calves.

With its ability to improve circulation, ginkgo is the premier plant medicine for intermittent claudication. It improves blood flow through the legs just as it does through the heart and brain by opening (dilating) the arteries.

Macular degeneration. Macular degeneration, a progressive, painless disorder, is the leading cause of legal blindness for the elderly of the United States. As eye cells break down, pigment and scar tissue accumulate in the center of the retina of the eye, causing a blind spot. Reading, driving, and even walking are impaired.

Ginkgo's strength in improving vision is its ability to fight the damage done by free radicals in the sensitive tissues of the retina. Ginkgo can also improve blood flow in the eye, where the retina demands a steady supply of glucose and oxygen.

In one six-month study, people who received 80 milligrams of a standardized ginkgo extract twice daily significantly improved their long-distance vision. Another study suggests that ginkgo extract may even reverse damage in the retina.

With my bilberry, ginkgo, and daily carrot to munch on, once again I have a triple whammy to slow down the ravages of maculitis, which recently led my first cousin Tom to surgery.

Migraines. Migraines are the Tyrannosaurus of headaches— there's almost no stopping them. Pain may be so severe that symptoms include nausea and vomiting.

Migraines are vascular headaches—that is, they are associated with the supply of blood to the brain. Ginkgo can improve blood flow to the brain, help maintain vascular tone, and keep blood vessels from leaking inflammatory chemicals. In one study, ginkgo reduced headaches in 80 percent of the long-term migraine sufferers who took it.

Tieraona Low Dog, M.D., is a family practice physician at the University of New Mexico Hospital, a professional member of the American Herbalists Guild, and a member of the Alternative Medicine Research Group at the University of New Mexico School of Medicine in Albuquerque. She acknowledges that ginkgo provides some people with relief from migraines.

Dr. Low Dog speculates that ginkgo's ability to improve cerebral circulation lessens initial vasoconstriction and consequent ischemia (blood deficiency) associated with migraines. Ginkgolides also act against the platelet activating factor, thus blocking inflammation and allergic responses. For whatever reason, ginkgo prevents migraines for some people.

Donald Brown, N.D., naturopathic physician and co-author of *The Natural Pharmacy*, recommends ginkgo for migraines if his patients do not respond first to the herb feverfew.

Raynaud's disease. This condition is similar to intermittent claudication, but it more often involves the hands, not the legs, and it is caused by poor blood flow brought on by cold temperatures and, sometimes, emotion. People suffering from Raynaud's frequently have frigid, stiff fingers, and it is more common among women than men.

Because there are ample European studies showing that ginkgo improves blood circulation, European physicians frequently prescribe it for Raynaud's. American doctors usually prescribe steroids, but I'd

 A CASE IN POINT

Taking a Longer Walk

In a study published in 1998, German researchers studied ginkgo's effect on patients suffering from two conditions: peripheral occlusive arterial disease, or a narrowing of blood vessels in the limbs, and intermittent claudication, or lameness.

At the start, all patients could walk little more than 100 meters without pain. Then, one group of patients was given ginkgo, and another group took a placebo.

After 24 weeks of regular walking, the ginkgo-taking patients clearly fared better. They increased their pain-free walking distance by about 50 percent. The placebo-taking control group, on the other hand, was able to walk only about 25 percent farther than when they started the study. The conclusions: Not only is ginkgo safe under these experimental conditions, but it helps such patients walk farther, pain-free.

rather try ginkgo instead of something that could have unpleasant side effects such as weight gain, acne, and irregular heartbeat.

Tinnitus. A constant ringing, buzzing, or whistling sound in the ears can be a problem for older people. Instead of responding to an outside stimulus, the acoustic nerve is triggered by something internal. Thought to be a result of poor circulation in the brain, tinnitus can be relieved by ginkgo.

In one European study in the mid-1980s, all patients taking 320 milligrams of ginkgo daily for a month improved much more than those taking a placebo.

Although some tinnitus sufferers have not been helped by ginkgo, Stephen Nagler, M.D., director of the Southeastern Comprehensive Tinnitus Clinic in Atlanta, says he expects some conclusive answers when the results of the first large-scale study on the effectiveness of ginkgo for tinnitus, being conducted at Birmingham University in the United Kingdom, are published in the near future.

How to Take It and How Much

I cannot endorse ingesting dry ginkgo leaves (even though I have personally consumed fresh leaves blended into fruit juice and even chewed one or two at a time), because the capsules contain the equivalent of 50 leaves per day. The leaves don't taste good and have never been considered foods, unlike more than half of Duke's Dozen.

Besides, fresh ginkgo leaves contain some unwanted substances that may cause allergic reactions. Ginkgolic acid is too closely related to urushiol, the chemical in poison ivy and poison oak that causes rashes. Germany now precludes sales of ginkgo products containing more than 5 ppm (parts per million) ginkgolic acid.

That's why I take my ginkgo in standardized capsule or liquid form, following label directions. Standardized products provide the same amount of active ingredients per dose. Look for ginkgo tablets that are standardized to contain 24 percent ginkgo flavonoid glycosides.

For most purposes, the usual dose is 120 milligrams of standardized extract per day, or one 40-milligram capsule taken three times a day with water at meals. Liquid extracts also are available. The standard dose is 30 to 60 drops three times a day.

During a trip to Belize, in Central America, a fellow traveler told me that he was getting very good relief from Raynaud's using a certain brand of ginkgo extract. A few days after switching brands, however, his hands went numb and cold while he was at the wheel of his car. Back in his office, he immediately started taking his former brand of ginkgo, and once again his symptoms were controlled. The moral of this story? Not all ginkgo products are alike. Go with the better standardized product, even if it costs more.

Useful Combinations

I like the idea of speeding the delivery of my food "farmaceuticals" to the brain via ginkgo's improved cerebral circulation.

Antioxidant foods. Many researchers now suspect that aging is just a lifetime's accumulation of oxidative damage, so I say the more antioxidants, the better. I try to eat all the richly-colored, antioxidant-rich foods I can—dark green, leafy vegetables, bright orange carrots and squash, and royal

DR. DUKE'S RECIPES

Cerebral Choline Chowder

All legumes are rich in choline, an important substance in brain and nerve tissue.

Select several of your favorites, such as black, adzuki, kidney, or lima beans; or black-eyed, chick-, split-, or field peas; plus lentils, if you like. Soak them overnight, then slowly simmer them the next day until tender with diced onion and garlic for flavor and for antioxidants.

Season your soup with fennel, rosemary, sage, savory, or thyme. All of these herbs have several compounds with the ability to slow the loss of choline, which is what U.S. Food and Drug Administration (FDA) approved synthetic Alzheimer's drugs do.

At the last minute of simmering, add some dandelion blossoms (up to 1 cup of flowers per each 2 cups of beans). You'll be taking one step toward a weed-free lawn (don't pick dandelion blossoms from a nonorganic yard) in addition to getting a good amount of choline-rich lecithin (nearly 3 percent on a dry weight basis). Lecithin contains choline. Lecithin is an important substance found in all cells and is involved in many vital functions, such as the liver's metabolism of fats, as well as the synthesis of new tissue.

purple bilberries, blueberries, grapes, and cherries. Then I take my ginkgo capsules at mealtimes like a good ol' boy.

And since Alzheimer's disease is also associated with low levels of acetylcholine, a substance in nerve cells that helps transmit impulses, I'll take my ginkgo with choline-rich bean soup to maximize its potential.

Caution: Contraindications, Interactions, and Side Effects

Compared to some synthetic drugs, ginkgo extract's side effects are minor and rare. According to the *Lawrence Review of Natural Products* and Volker Schulz, Rudolf Hansel, and Varro E. Tyler's book *Rational Phytotherapy—A Physician's Guide to Herbal Medicine,* ginkgo's adverse effects can include allergic dermatitis, anxiety, diarrhea, gastrointestinal upset, headache, insomnia, and nausea.

Pharmaceutical alert. More serious, at least for those on blood thinners like Coumadin, is that ginkgo, like garlic, can slow blood's ability to clot. Taking one or both of these herbs in conjunction with anticoagulant drugs could be dangerous.

DR. DUKE'S NOTES

The first green sprout to appear in Hiroshima after the atomic bomb was that of a ginkgo tree. Ginkgo even survives in New York City.

Dr. Nagler recommends that people taking ginkgo for more than three months also take a simple, painless "bleeding time" test to measure coagulation time. Warning signs that ginkgo is interfering with platelet aggregation might include bleeding gums, nosebleeds, or bruising, he says. Dr. Nagler cites a report in the June 1996 issue of *Neurology* of a woman who experienced serious internal bleeding after taking ginkgo for two years in conjunction with no other drugs but acetaminophen, the active ingredient in Tylenol.

Also, do not use ginkgo if you are also taking antidepressant monoamine oxidase inhibitor drugs such as phenelzine sulfate (Nardil) or tranylcypromine (Parnate), aspirin, or other nonsteroidal anti-inflammatory medications.

Allergy alert. Though ginkgo is regarded by many as a poisonous plant, some experts insist there is not sufficient accumulated data to support this. I cannot give the fruit pulp, leaves, or even the edible seed a clean bill of health. Clearly, its bilobin and ginkgolic acid are similar to poison ivy's active irritating ingredient. Touching the pulp of the ginkgo fruit frequently results in a rash, and it's also possible that ginkgo leaves could cause an allergic reaction in some susceptible people.

Toxicity. Too many of the edible seeds can cause serious problems, even death. I've read reports of children who have died after eating only seven seeds. The Chinese boil the seeds to remove the toxins, but I don't recommend that anyone experiment with this.

chapter nine

Hawthorn

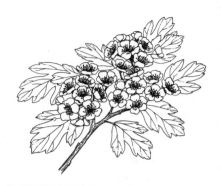

LATIN NAME: *Crataegus monogyna*
FAMILY NAME: Rosaceae

MY GENES REQUIRE that I put certain herbs at the top of my herbal hit parade. I take celery seed to prevent the gout that plagues all the Duke boys, myself included. I take echinacea and garlic as a precaution against colon cancer, which killed my father and two uncles.

But there's no history of heart disease in my family tree, so it may seem odd that I rank hawthorn high in the pantheon of Duke's Dozen. My wife Peggy, on the other hand, *does* have a genetic predisposition to heart disease, since both of her parents suffered heart problems. At first glance, hawthorn probably belongs more in her medicine chest than mine.

But after mulling it over, I decided to add hawthorn to my list of essential herbs. You see, my genes alone don't tell the whole story. Unlike my parents, I smoked like a chimney—three packs a day for nearly 30 years. Even though I kicked the habit way back in 1971, I'm sure the smoking took its toll on my lungs and heart. Good genes or not, a heart attack may be on the horizon.

Add to that the stress of day-to-day living. Even though I'm retired, I'm probably under more stress now than in all the years I worked as a botanist for the U.S. Department of Agriculture. I'm always under the pressure of writing deadlines (this book was no exception), and I give over 200 lectures a year. Racing to the airport, then to the hotel, then to the lecture hall, and then back again to the airport sure takes a toll on the ticker.

My trips to the Amazon aren't stress-free, either. Heat, frustration, overexertion, and local political problems all combine to create conditions ripe for a coronary. Add to that my penchant for adventure, like the time I ignored my shaman's advice and waded through knee-deep waters in a flooded black lagoon. Electric eels, stingrays, and anacondas lurked below the surface. Just sharing the same space with an anaconda is enough to bring on heart failure.

But whenever I visit my doctor, he doesn't seem concerned. My electrocardiograms (EKGs) have never raised so much as an eyebrow, let alone an alarm. Still, an ounce of hawthorn is worth a pound of cure. It's loaded with heart-smart oligomeric procyanidins (OPCs) and bioflavonoids, which can help keep your heart rhythm regular and prevent a variety of heart problems. I take hawthorn anytime my stress levels are elevated. And I'd take it religiously if I had a mild heart condition.

What Hawthorn Is and What It Can Do

Hawthorn in a deciduous flowering shrub with small thorns, stocky branches, and small, red, oval fruits that look a lot like crabapples. You'll find it residing along roadsides, in fields, and in wooded areas throughout Europe and in parts of North America, mainly in the Northeast but also south beyond the Carolinas and west at least as far as Oklahoma. The hawthorn bush can soar as high as 40 feet.

DR. DUKE'S NOTES

Hawthorn is often grown as an ornamental hedge in England.

There are at least 200 species of hawthorn, and I don't know a trained botanist—let alone a gardener, herbalist, chemist, pharmacist, or physician—who can tell them apart.

The fruit is tart to the taste. I sampled several species last year at the Colonial Garden in Plymouth, Massachusetts, and I've tried even tastier fruit at the Coker Arboretum at my alma mater, the University of North Carolina. Native Americans ate many species of *Crataegus*. Today, though, naturopathic physicians usually don't recommend eating the wild fruit raw. While I consider them food plants and eat them raw and fresh—in moderation—any time I come across one that tastes good, I can't endorse the practice for anyone else (except for close family and friends). A safer bet is to eat the fruit dried or cooked, perhaps as a jelly. The fruit can also be brewed into a heady wine, and its young leaves and white flowers steeped to make a tea. Interestingly, hawthorn contains many of the same compounds as common teas, including black, green, and oolong teas, promoted these days for a variety of health benefits. But the standardized capsule is what I recommend for heart health.

Help for Your Heart

Germany's prestigious Commission E, a panel of experts roughly equivalent to the U.S. Food and Drug Administration, has approved hawthorn for a number of heart problems. It's widely used in Europe for treating angina, which causes chest pains and is brought on by blockage in the arteries. Varro E. Tyler, Ph.D., Sc.D., professor emeritus of pharmacognosy at Perdue University, discusses hawthorn's heart-health benefits in his excellent book, *Herbs of Choice*. The OPCs in hawthorn, he explains, have beta-blocking activities. (Beta-blockers are drugs prescribed to increase coronary blood flow and help lower blood pressure and heart rate, stopping arrhythmias.) Hawthorn also contains flavonoids, compounds that open up the coronary arteries. It appears to stabilize heart rhythm, decrease palpitations brought on by anxiety, increase exercise tolerance, reduce blood pressure, and lower cholesterol levels. In their book *The Natural Pharmacy*, Skye W. Lininger and his colleagues say that hawthorn "may" improve blood flow through the coronary arteries.

Because hawthorn is a powerful heart medication, I'd advise erring on the side of caution. Literature from some leading British and

Modern science validates hawthorn's centuries-old use as an effective means of strengthening the heart and staving off cardiac problems. Hawthorn activity is due primarily to proanthocyanidins and flavonoids, including quercetin, hyperoside, vitexin, vitexin-rhamnoside, and rutin. Flavonoids are a large class of pigments found in plants that protect blood vessels, aid in circulation, stimulate bile production, and lower cholesterol levels. Proanthocyanidins are one of 12 classes of flavonoids. Oligomeric proanthocyanidins (OPCs) are one type of proanthocyanidin. The cardioprotective effects of proanthocyanidins have been supported by recent studies of red wine and grape seeds.

German research scientists suggests that hawthorn is not suitable for self-medication. True! No one should try to treat a serious heart condition on his or her own. Before you take hawthorn, talk to your doctor. But I do recommend the tasty species as a preventive food for the strong of heart.

How Hawthorn Can Help

Hawthorn can be used to treat a variety of health problems and, according to European clinical experience, is safe to use over extended periods of time. Here are some of the conditions for which it's shown to be effective:

Good Heart Health

Hawthorn seems to be helpful for a variety of cardiac problems.

Angina pectoris. Caused by a deficient blood supply to the heart, symptoms of angina include tightness, pressure, or burning in the chest, and pain that may radiate to the left shoulder, down the left arm, and to the back or jaw. Exercise can exacerbate the problem, since it puts extra pressure on the arteries as they try to deliver more oxygen-rich blood to the muscles. Similarly, stress, fear, and anger all get the heart pumping faster, and they too can bring on angina.

The nutrients magnesium and niacin, found in fruits and vegetables including hawthorn, have been long recommended for treating angina. People deficient in these nutrients can get them from hawthorn and other supplements. Research supports the use of hawthorn for treating angina. In their book, *Herbal Medicines: A Guide for Healthcare Professionals*, authors Carol Newall, Linda Anderson, and J. David Phillipson report that German researchers gave 60 angina patients 60 milligrams of hawthorn three times daily, with positive results.

Arrhythmia. Cardiac arrhythmia is an irregular beating of the heart. If the heart races more than 100 beats per minute, the condition is called tachycardia. A heartbeat slower than 60 beats per minute is known as bradycardia. Abnormal heart rhythm can result in atrial arrhythmia, a "pooling" of blood if the heart can't pump it from its upper chambers, which can lead to clotting, heart attack, or stroke. Ventricular arrhythmia affects the lower chambers in the heart, leading to ventricular fibrillation, a condition in which the heart flutters weakly instead of pumping powerfully. A significant number of fatal heart attacks are attributed to ventricular fibrillation.

Studies have shown that hawthorn extracts administered to rabbits have a beneficial effect on arrhythmia. I've heard one report that hawthorn can induce arrhythmias, but I don't put much stock in this single, isolated finding. A single reported case just doesn't win the race! Still, it's advisable to check with your doctor.

Atherosclerosis. This heart condition results when cholesterol, lipids, and calcium deposits clog the arteries. It's the most common form of arteriosclerosis, in which vessels become diseased—they thicken, harden, and lose elasticity. Arteriosclerosis is a leading cause of death in the United States, and family history isn't the only determining factor in developing this condition. A sedentary lifestyle, high cholesterol, obesity, cigarette smoking, and stress all play a part.

While you can't change your genes, you *can* change your lifestyle. Call a halt to bad habits, get off your duff and exercise, and eat a heart-healthy diet full of OPC-laden fruits, including dried or cooked hawthorn, prunes, strawberries, rosehips, peaches, crabapples, pears, and blackberries. All are members of the rose family, along with cherries, plums, chokecherries, wineberries, cloudberries, and apricots.

Doctors often recommend aspirin, a blood thinner, to prevent a second heart attack. Hawthorn, too, has blood-thinning properties—in fact, it reportedly contains at least seven known blood thinners.

Cardiovascular insufficiency. This is a broad term for the inadequate performance of the heart and blood vessels. People who have it report reduced performance in cardiovascular activities, shortness of breath, and swelling of the ankles. In one German study, researchers treated 136 patients with cardiovascular insufficiency and found that their condition improved, with minimal risk.

Dyspnea. Breathing difficulty and chest pain can be caused by circulation disturbances or blood that lacks sufficient oxygen. According to *Potter's New Cyclopaedia of Botanical Drugs and Preparations*, clinical trials in Japan showed that 80 patients given hawthorn fruits and leaves showed improvement in dyspnea, edema, and cardiac function.

Edema. Edema causes bloating, swelling, and inflammation among patients with heart problems, which is one reason why diuretics are often prescribed for heart patients.

Hawthorn is blessed with at least nine antiedemics. In *Herbal Medicinals: A Clinician's Guide*, Miller and Murray share an interesting case study of a 62-year-old man with congestive heart failure. An herbalist recommended that he take hawthorn, which reportedly lessened his edema and improved his physical endurance.

High blood pressure. Hawthorn contains at least three antihypertensives, which help keep blood pressure from rising. Lucinda G. Miller, Pharm.D., and Wallace Murray, authors of *Herbal Medicinals: A Clinician's Guide* report that hawthorn expands blood vessels, lowering blood pressure and reducing the heart's workload.

High cholesterol. High cholesterol can lead to serious complications including cardiovascular disease, a major health problem in the United States responsible for the most deaths, the largest number of hospitalizations, and the greatest number of pharmaceutical prescriptions. The best way to prevent heart problems, of course, is to keep your heart strong and healthy with regular exercise and a low-fat, low-cholesterol diet.

I would also look to hawthorn. A study from the biochemistry department at the University of Madras, India, shows that a tincture of hawthorn berries can help ward off high blood cholesterol and atherosclerosis.

Attention-Deficit Hyperactivity Disorder

While hawthorn is best-known as a heart-helper, there is some indication that it may be useful in treating attention-deficit hyperactivity disorder (ADHD), a condition marked by an inability to stay focused and attentive, and a particular problem among children. David Winston, a noted East Coast herbalist, tells me that he uses hawthorn not only for heart problems but also for ADHD. While he prefers to work with a solid extract of the fruit of the European species, *Crataegus monogyna*, he says he's happy with any of the native American species that have white flowers, believing them to be almost as effective as European hawthorns. He believes these flowers have even more biologically active effects than the fruits. His "Focus Formula" for ADHD

A CASE IN POINT

Hawthorn Successes

I've heard many success stories from people who've tried hawthorn. Here are two:

Christopher Hobbs, author of *Handmade Medicines*, recently told me about his father, Ken, a botanist and former university professor. Ken had a massive heart attack when he was 48 years old. During his recovery, he started taking hawthorn, and his doctor was amazed at his progress. Today, Ken is 78 and still takes hawthorn faithfully. His circulation has improved, and his heart is strong and steady.

And a registered nurse who's a frequent guest on my Peruvian eco-tours told me that hawthorn changed her family's life. She has weaned her husband off his heart medication and put him on hawthorn and linden instead. She persuaded her father to take hawthorn for cardiomyopathy. And she recommended hawthorn as a natural diuretic to her younger sister, who has insulin-dependent diabetes and suffered an allergic reaction to a prescription diuretic.

includes oats, fresh lemon balm, dried hawthorn fruit and flower, dried autumn ginkgo leaf, and fresh skullcap herb.

The drug Ritalin is widely prescribed to treat ADHD in children—far too widely, in my opinion. Instead, I'd try making a hawthorn sauce, just as I'd make an applesauce, and spice it up with cinnamon. I'll bet that kids like it better.

How to Take It and How Much

Hawthorn is available in several forms: fresh, dried, liquid extracts, tinctures, powders, and capsules. I think everyone should make the fruit part of a healthy diet, in cooked or dried form—not raw (even though I eat it raw). Our hungrier ancestors probably ate any ripe hawthorn berry they encountered. If you take the dried fruit, a suggested dosage is 0.3 to 1 gram per day.

Standardized extracts of hawthorn, in my view, may be taken by people with minor heart problems, but let me reiterate: Talk to your doctor before you take hawthorn. It's very important that you take the right kind of standardized extract at the appropriate daily dosage, extracts containing 1.8 percent vitexin-4-rhamnosides or 10 percent OPCs in dosages of 120 to 240 milligrams three times per day.

Useful Combinations

Naturopaths and nutritionists often recommend other heart-wise herbs, vitamins, and nutrients along with hawthorn.

Angelica. Calcium deposits in the arteries can lead to heart complications. Angelica can help. This natural calcium antagonist reportedly contains at least 15 calcium-blocking compounds. Two have been shown to have better calcium-fighting functions that Verapamil, an angina medication.

This kind of data prompted me to cook up a concoction called "Angelade." The primary ingredient is juiced angelica, along with other foods that contain calcium blockers including carrot, celery, fennel, parsley, and parsnip (for the recipe, see page 75).

Animal musk. My good friends Albert Leung, Ph.D., and nationally known herbalist Steven Foster, authors of several useful books including my favorite, *Encyclopedia of Common Natural Ingredients,* report that clinical trials of musk in China showed improvement in about 74 percent of heart patients—a track record as good or better than the prescription medication nitroglycerin. To clarify: This is animal musk, not the vegetable musks from the mallow family. As an herbalist, I don't work with musk myself.

Celery juice. Tip back a cold glass of celery juice. In one study of rats fed a high-fat diet for eight weeks, those given a celery juice supplement showed lowered total cholesterol, LDL, and triglycerides, a fatty substance in the blood that is also an important factor in the development of heart disease. Clinical trials in the United States showed that the equivalent of four stalks of celery lowered blood pressure.

Pineapple enzyme. California herbalist Kathi Keville, whom I greatly admire, says that more than 400 research papers—most of them from Germany—have been devoted to the medicinal uses of bromelain, an enzyme found in pineapple. One such study, done in the early 1970s, showed that angina patients who took bromelain enjoyed relief from their symptoms within 4 to 90 days, depending on the seriousness of their condition. Their heart problems returned when they stopped taking the enzyme.

Walnuts. Walnuts and other nuts high in monounsaturated fatty acids, such as almonds, filberts, macadamias, pistachios, pecans, and

 HERB LORE AND MORE

Hawthorn has a long history as a heart tonic in herbal folklore. Europeans, Chinese, and Native American peoples used the herb as a cardiac medication, brewed as a tea or taken in tincture form. The Cherokees also used an infusion of the bark to prevent heart spasms.

Besides heart conditions, hawthorn tea was also taken to soothe sore throats and as a natural diuretic for kidney disorders. Native Americans often treated rheumatism with hawthorn, and its flowers and berries were gathered for their astringent properties.

Today, traditional Chinese practitioners still use hawthorn as an aid in the digestion of fatty foods.

the delicious avocado fruit, may lower cholesterol, helping to keep the heart strong. Research has shown that a diet with 20 percent of calories from walnuts lowered total cholesterol by 12 percent and low-density lipoprotein (LDL), often called "bad cholesterol," by 16 percent.

Herbal combination. Dr. Leung and Foster also suggest Canada balsam, cassia, cinnamon, and turmeric (for more information on turmeric, see chapter 15) for heart and chest pain.

Nutrient combination. Studies support a combination of four nutrients to treat heart disease: I-carnitine, Coenzyme Q_{10}, magnesium, and vitamin E. A suggested preventive dose is 1,000 milligrams per day of I-carnitine, 100 milligrams of CoQ_{10}, 800 milligrams of magnesium, and 800 IU (international units) of vitamin E. Supplements are recommended, since it's tough to get these levels even from eating the best of my plants.

Caution: Contraindications, Interactions, and Side Effects

Hawthorn is considered extremely safe even when used over long periods of time. For the most part (with the exception noted below), there are no known interactions with prescription heart medications or other types of drugs. Still, it bears repeating that you should consult your doctor before using hawthorn, and keep the following possible side effects in mind.

Fatigue. Known but rarely reported side effects of hawthorn include fatigue, possibly accompanied by nausea, rash, and sweating.

Depression. Flower extracts may act as a mild depressant.

Pregnancy alert. I always caution that all medicines, both herbal and pharmaceutical, be avoided unless approved by your obstetrician. Having said that, I wouldn't discourage my own pregnant daughter from using hawthorn in food form—cautiously—if she had a heart condition. I'd also suggest other members of the rose family, including apples and crabapples, as they're almost certainly safer than prescription drugs.

Pharmaceutical alert. Studies suggest that in the early stages of heart disease, hawthorn is more effective than the commonly prescribed digitalis, a drug derived from the herb foxglove, and has fewer side effects. However, if you're on digitalis, you should never try hawthorn or any herbal medication without consulting your doctor. Hawthorn may make digitalis more active.

 ## A CASE IN POINT

The Frantic Father

The caller sounded desperately worried. He had a question about using hawthorn for cardiac arrhythmia, a condition in which the heart beats irregularly, typically racing ahead or skipping a beat. Cardiac arrhythmias can lead to potentially fatal heart attacks.

I expected him to tell me that he himself had been diagnosed with the condition, which usually occurs in adults over age 50. But he explained that the person with the problem was his little girl, only 6 years old.

Calcium channel-blockers—the medication customarily prescribed for this condition—weren't working for his daughter, he told me. My first thought was, "Oh no! He's going to ask me to prescribe an herbal medication over the phone." This is something I never do—and I'd certainly never reconsider in a condition as serious as a cardiac disorder in a child. To my relief, he wasn't looking for an herbal prescription. His daughter's doctor, he said, had already turned to the alternative medicine chest, suggesting a regimen including hawthorn, Coenzyme Q_{10}, and magnesium. Research has shown that all three help the heart.

The alternative approach, the father reported, was working for his young daughter. But he was concerned about hawthorn's toxic effects if used over a long period of time. I scoured my herbal database, reviewed the literature, and faxed him all the evidence I could muster. Turns out, hawthorn seems to be safe even for long-term use. I found no links between hawthorn and heart attacks. I did find one isolated report to the effect that hawthorn can induce arrhythmias, and I felt obligated to tell him about it, but I frankly don't place too much stock in it.

If it were my daughter, I sure would rather give her hawthorn than a pharmaceutically synthetic calcium channel-blocker. It certainly worked for my caller, since his daughter got better.

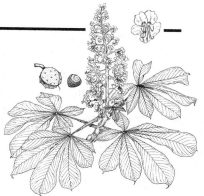

chapter ten

Horse Chestnut

LATIN NAME: *Aesculus hippocastanum*
FAMILY NAME: Hippocastanaceae

AS A BOY GROWING UP around Raleigh, North Carolina, I loved to forage through the woods and wetlands for all manner of treasures from the wild. Sometimes I went alone, and sometimes with friends. But always, when we passed the native American horse chestnut trees (buckeyes) growing on the margins of the swamps and the European horse chestnuts cultivated there, we would pocket the shiny brown nuts. Legend was they would bring us good luck. And we believed.

Some 60 years later, as an adult living in Maryland, I'm still not sure where the horse chestnut got its reputation for good fortune. Maybe it worked, though. I'm still going strong. And my many years as a botanist have taken me, sometimes fortuitously, around the globe to learn about plants.

In recent years, I've learned a lot more about the horse chestnut, too. It is renowned for its value as a medicinal herb, especially by Europeans, who use it topically and internally to prevent and treat varicose veins and other peripheral vascular conditions.

My wife, Peg, and I both suffer from vascular problems now that we're seniors. Incidence seems to increase with age. I have a number of unsightly spiderlike lines called telangiectases. Peg is more bothered by edema in her legs and the blue rivulets so characteristic of varicose veins.

Peg has gone the traditional route recently, buying expensive compression stockings to help with circulation. But I'm looking to my six-acre herbal vineyard, where I grow an American relative of the native European horse chestnut. I don't pluck the nuts for medicinal purposes. Rather, I cultivate the tree to teach others about the herb—and to remind myself to take the standardized capsules I keep in the house.

Have they worked for me? My spider veins are still there, but I haven't developed varicose veins or chronic venous insufficiency, a condition that causes swelling, aches, and fatigue in the legs. I think horse chestnut is helping me stave them off.

Recently, I ordered an *Aesculus hippocastanum* tree from Europe, which I will add to my garden. I probably won't crush its nuts to make medicine. Standardized formulas simply are more reliable. But I may put one in my pocket.

What Horse Chestnut Is and What It Can Do

Aesculus hippocastanum is a tall tree native to Albania, Bulgaria, Greece, and Yugoslavia. It is widely cultivated elsewhere, especially in western Europe. In the newsletter *Alternative Medicine Alert*, Philippe O. Szapary and Michael D. Cirigliano, both M.D.'s, say the European species was introduced to the United States as a shade tree in 1740.

It has pretty white flowers and leaves that are digitate. If you put out your hand and spread your fingers, you get an idea of the leaves' shape. The nuts, about an inch or two in diameter, are peeled and mashed for their pulp, which is rich in bioactive ingredients. The bark, flowers, and leaves also contain medicinal properties.

A European Nut of Choice

To my knowledge, only the European horse chestnut has been studied for its medicinal value, mostly by the Germans and the

French. Of 12 other varieties, seven are native to the United States—including the well-known Ohio buckeye—and five to India and Asia. I have found no solid studies to show whether any of the dozen contain the same phytochemicals or produce similar responses.

The European nut is high in aescin, a compound that builds up vein walls, and rutin, which helps maintain the integrity of capillaries. Aescin and rutin work synergistically with other active chemicals to reduce inflammation and pain and improve circulation. That's why horse chestnut is in Duke's Dozen.

If you've never heard of horse chestnut, or haven't heard much, that's probably because it's just gaining attention in the United States. People often are surprised when I tell them that horse chestnut is a medicinal plant. Like me, many learned as children that the nut is poisonous. I think its toxic nature may have been exaggerated, although it may be mildly poisonous if high quantities are ingested before processing.

Unlike the sweet chestnut—no relation and actually from the oak family—the somewhat bitter-tasting horse chestnut is not considered a food plant. But in some countries, horse chestnut is being made into flour as a source of edible starches. A 1996 issue of the Italian journal

FROM MY SCIENCE NOTEBOOK

First, a mini refresher course: Arteries are the main tubes in our bodies that carry oxygen-rich blood away from the heart. Veins are vessels that move blood back to the heart, and capillaries connect the two.

Most studies on horse chestnut have focused on the herb as a treatment for vascular conditions, in which the capillaries are weak or the veins are not working properly. With varicose veins, for example, the weakened veins may bulge and leak blood that forms pools under the skin, creating those tortuous blue lines, itching, fatigue, and discomfort in the legs.

The European horse chestnut contains many active compounds that help fight inflammation, edema, pain, and the weakening of veins and capillaries. Perhaps most important are rutin, which helps strengthen fragile capillaries, and aescin (sometimes spelled escin), which inhibits enzymes that damage the interiors of the veins.

dedicated to the study of medicinal plants, *Fitoterapia*, notes that the scientific name *Aesculus* means nutrient, or edible.

I think standardized formulas are quite safe, although I strongly advise against crushing and nibbling the unprocessed nuts. There is still some controversy about whether the raw nuts are edible. Play it safe and don't experiment with questionable plants.

Commission E (a German panel of experts roughly equivalent to the U.S. Food and Drug Administration) approves standardized horse chestnut for treatment of pathological conditions of the veins of the legs, including pain and a sensation of heaviness, nocturnal cramping of the calves, pruritis, and swelling. Along with many herbalists, I interpret that to include varicose and spider veins, within the broad definition of chronic venous insufficiency.

Today, horse chestnut is popular throughout Europe for the treatment and prevention of those conditions, and for hemorrhoids— which are no more than varicose veins of the anus and rectum. Ointments containing horse chestnut also are used to soothe sports injuries, such as strains and sprains. Some research indicates that horse chestnut may even be valuable in the treatment of wrinkles, hair loss, cellulite, backache, and arthritis.

How Horse Chestnut Can Help

Horse chestnut has a variety of popular applications. Here are some of the best documented:

Hemorrhoids. These swollen veins of the anus and lower rectum stretch under pressure, sometimes causing pain, itching, and the appearance of bright red blood on the stool or toilet paper, the National Digestive Diseases Information Clearinghouse reports.

Hemorrhoids are common, especially during pregnancy, because of pressure from the fetus, says the clearinghouse, an office of the NIH.

Other potential causes include chronic diarrhea or constipation and straining to have a bowel movement, it says. About half of women and men get hemorrhoids by age 50. For some, the condition is hereditary.

Traditional treatments include warm baths, ice packs, hemorrhoidal creams or suppositories, and regular consumption of dietary fiber and nonalcoholic beverages. Sometimes, hemorrhoids must be treated surgically, says the NIH.

One of the earliest studies on horse chestnut, done way back in 1896, demonstrated its usefulness in treating hemorrhoids, using an alcoholate of the nut to show its anesthetic and anti-inflammatory activity in treating varicosis, in general, and hemorrhoids, in particular. More than a century later, Europeans are still convinced. Many reach for standardized horse chestnut to treat hemorrhoids. I'd try it too, if I had this condition.

Varicose veins (and other peripheral vascular conditions). The tortuous blue varicose veins that appear just under the skin, most often in the leg below the knee, are easy to spot. Too easy, for many who suffer from them.

Not only do varicose veins look unattractive, but they can throb,

 HERB LORE AND MORE

Traditionally, the bark of *Aesculus hippocastanum* has been used as a tonic, narcotic, and febrifuge, according to information collected by British herbalist Maude Grieve. Folklore has it that the fruit and other plant parts were used to treat backache, bruises, cough, diarrhea, dysentery, menstrual discomfort, eczema, phlebitis, thrombophlebitis, and gastrosis.

Native Americans picked up on the transplanted horse chestnut's medicinal value. The Iroquois used a compound of the powdered root to treat chest pain, according to James William Herrick, author of *Iroquois Medical Botany*. The Shinnecocks and Mohegans carried the horse chestnut in their pockets as a treatment for rheumatism, note Lloyd G. Carr and Carlos Westey, in a 1945 *Journal of American Folklore*. Maybe that's the origin of the good-luck tale that led my boyhood friends and me to pocket fallen horse chestnuts.

itch, cramp, ache, burn, and feel heavy and uncomfortable, according to the National Heart, Lung, and Blood Institute, an office of the National Institutes of Health (NIH). The legs may swell, too; varicose means "swollen."

Varicose veins sometimes run in families. They may be aggravated by excess weight, hormonal changes such as pregnancy, or tight clothing that limits circulation, the NIH says. Women experience them more often than do men.

Normally, oxygen-carrying blood travels through our veins, back to the heart. Valves in the veins keep blood from flowing backward. When the valves don't work or are weak, blood pools in our veins, the NIH says. These pools stretch the veins, which become swollen.

There is no cure for varicose veins. Exercise helps boost circulation, while elevating the legs during rest relieves discomfort, the NIH says. Women can wear support or compression stockings, as Peg did for a while, to help push blood toward the heart. Other traditional options include surgery, injecting a solution to diminish the veins or zapping them with lasers for cosmetic improvement.

With spider veins, compression is standard treatment, although a solution also can be injected to eliminate them.

I'll reach for horse chestnut before trying expensive cosmetic treatments.

A study out of West Germany, reported in the early 1980s, showed one commercial horse chestnut product affected both the collagen content and architecture of the varicose vein and helped make the veins more normal.

Horse chestnut may also relieve symptoms of chronic venous insufficiency (CVI), which sometimes leads to varicose veins. Symptoms of CVI include edema, enlarged veins near the skin surface, and fatigue in the legs. Standing or walking aggravates symptoms. Sitting and elevating the feet usually helps.

Sometimes, my legs ache after I've been on them a while. I exercise to build muscle and improve my circulation, but I want to do all that I can to prevent CVI. That's another reason I supplement with horse chestnut. And the science is in my corner. Denise Webb, Ph.D., an associate editor of *Environmental Nutrition* newsletter, reported on a review of 13 studies on horse chestnut for CVI that showed the seed extract worked better than a placebo and as well as standard medications at reducing symptoms.

How to Take It and How Much

A few years ago, it was hard to find horse chestnut in the United States. Now, capsules and tinctures are readily available. At least one supplement containing the seed extract is marketed on U.S. television. Ointments, too, are becoming easier to buy as this medicinal plant gains acceptance in America. Here are suggested uses, based on my research and experience.

 A CASE IN POINT

Kathleen's Story

Kathleen D., a schoolteacher living in Virginia, recently decided to fight varicose veins with standardized horse chestnut capsules.

A few years ago, Kathleen spent about $800 to have some bulging purple lines on her lower legs removed by the injection of a solution to diminish them. Now, she has a few more unsightly lines. She wants to get rid of them without spending a lot of money.

She had read about horse chestnut's anti-inflammatory and capillary-building attributes and its potential for preventing varicose veins. Even though Kathleen already takes a prescription diuretic for high blood pressure and an over-the-counter antihistamine for allergies, she was comfortable with adding horse chestnut to her regimen.

Kathleen purchased a bottle of standardized, 400-milligram capsules, which she now takes daily. It's too early to tell if horse chestnut will help her stave off varicose veins. "But I feel that it's safe," she says, "and worth a try."

Hemorrhoids. Again, an ointment may be used topically to treat swelling, pain, and itching. You also can use standardized tinctures or capsules, following the directions on the label. I think it would be safe—if not doubly effective—to use both.

You might even add Hoffman's infusion (below), drinking it or applying it topically. He recommends it for hemorrhoids, too.

Varicose veins, spider veins, and CVI. Buy standardized capsules and tinctures and follow label directions. I try to take four capsules a day, although sometimes I miss. My standardized 257-milligram capsules contain 18 to 27 percent aescin.

Most studies have looked at the plant's use internally. But there is some evidence that applying an ointment to the affected area may help, too. Why not try both?

David Hoffman, a British-trained medical herbalist, author of several good books including *The Herbal Handbook*, and an authority I respect, recommends making an infusion, if you can find the dried fruit. Pour boiling water onto 1 or 2 teaspoonfuls and let it infuse for about 15 minutes. Drink three times daily for varicosities, or apply it as a lotion.

Useful Combinations

Here are some remedies you can try, with or without standardized horse chestnut.

Butcher's broom and buckwheat. Both contain rutin, the same capillary-protector that's in horse chestnut. Buckwheat is made into a flour typically sold as a pancake mix. Both are marketed as extracts and teas for treating varicose veins.

Compression stockings. You don't have to give up on conventional therapies. Studies show that wearing compression stockings or support hose can help lessen symptoms of varicose veins by keeping the blood flowing toward the heart. Commission E recommends using support hose or other treatments prescribed by your doctor, along with horse chestnut.

Exercise. I've chosen gardening and walking for my moderate ex-

WHAT NEW RESEARCH TELLS US

Here's what we're learning about some exciting new possibilities for horse chestnut. Keep in mind that research is still in process.

Sports injuries. Some research indicates that horse chestnut ointments and lotions applied topically may help reduce the inflammation and pain of injuries, such as strains and sprains. "Numerous clinical studies and published case reports confirm the efficacy of aescin-containing topical products" for bruises, edema, fractures, sports injuries, sprains, and tendinitis, report Albert Leung, Ph.D., a pharmacognistic consultant, and Steven Foster, an herbalist, in their *Encyclopedia of Common Natural Ingredients*. They report numerous clinical and case studies looking at aescin-containing topical products. This is a popular use in Europe.

Hair loss. Is it horse chestnut or horse manure? Aesculin, one of many bioactives in horse chestnut, may help reduce hair loss when combined with ximenynic and lauric acids, according to three Italian researchers who reported their study of horse chestnut in *Fitoterapia* in 1996. A formula containing all three was applied to the scalps of males and females in a placebo-controlled study. It produced favorable effects on scalp microcirculation, they report. So would a shampoo and a massage, I suspect. We'll have to wait and see.

Cellulite. Apparently because of its strengthening effect on capillaries, horse chestnut extracts—and its active compounds, including aescin—are moving into the cosmetic field, especially in Europe. The same Italian research team reported that topical applications may help lessen the appearance of the unattractive dimples and lumps that plague thighs, bellies, and derrieres.

Wrinkles. Horse chestnut contains antioxidants that researchers believe may diminish the appearance of wrinkles, and at least one research report says the antioxidants have been shown to protect against ultraviolet damage to the skin. I haven't read the details, but I have applied the fruit to my face, hoping to lessen my lines. So far, the same 70-year-old is looking back in my mirror.

ercise program. They give me a chance to enjoy nature. Whatever forms you choose, exercise will help build muscle, improve circulation, and keep down your weight—all preventive strategies for peripheral vascular problems. It will help diminish symptoms, too.

Ginkgo. In addition to improving memory, ginkgo boosts circulation. Extracts have been promoted lately as topical agents, which may help prevent or ease varicose and spider veins, CVI, and even hemorrhoids. Perhaps ginkgo would help me remember to take my horse chestnut.

 # ALL IN THE FAMILY: BUTCHER'S BROOM

I'm going to blur family lines a bit here, because I want to also tell you about butcher's broom (and buckwheat—see page 168) for treating varicose veins and some other venous conditions. Butcher's broom isn't truly related to horse chestnut, from a taxonomist's point of view. But both are high in rutin.

Over the years, my wife, Peg, has spent hundreds of dollars on those high-priced compression stockings to ameliorate symptoms of edema and varicose veins. But I think she's finally thrown in the nylon; she doesn't buy them anymore.

I thought I had her hooked on horse chestnut a while back. She bought a bottle of standardized capsules but didn't stick with them. She is less persistent than I am and a much greater believer in pharmaceuticals. Perhaps I'll try to entice her with herbs once again, now that I'm cultivating butcher's broom in my garden. The herb, native to the Mediterranean, is part of my arsenal against varicose veins.

What Butcher's Broom Is and What It Can Do

Butcher's broom is a shrub, with small, spearlike leaves and red berries that resemble tiny cherry tomatoes. It sometimes is grown as an ornamental hedge. The young shoots reportedly have been eaten as asparagus and the matured branches were gathered and bound and sold as the name butcher's broom implies—for sweeping.

These days, butcher's broom is commonly used in Europe to treat hemorrhoids and varicose veins and other peripheral vascular conditions, inter-

A high-fiber diet. Eating lots of fiber—fruits, vegetables, and whole grains—along with plenty of nonalcoholic beverages, such as juice and water, lessens your chances of becoming constipated, a condition that contributes to hemorrhoids.

Violets and pansies. I used to pick violets and pansies—edible sources of rutin—from my garden and eat them as part of my strategy to prevent CVI and spider and varicose veins. I calculated I would need about 1 large pansy or 10 violets to get all the rutin I need. If you're foraging in your own backyard, that's about 100 Johnny-

nally and topically. It is sold as standardized capsules and tinctures and can be found in ointments and teas.

How Butcher's Broom Can Help

In addition to rutin, other active compounds called ruscogenins decrease swelling. So butcher's broom may help diminish those bulging blue lines in our lower legs.

Germany's Commission E approves butcher's broom as supportive therapy for CVI and hemorrhoids.

Krista Thie, a botanist in Washington state, tells me she uses butcher's broom for varicose veins. "It reduces pressure and itchiness and achiness," she says.

Useful Combinations

Donald Brown, N.D., editor of the *Quarterly Review of Natural Medicine*, suggests that health care professionals turn to butcher's broom in combination with horse chestnut seed extract to treat early stages of chronic venous insufficiency.

I may just add the butcher's broom shoots and seeds from my Green Farmacy Garden to my "rutinade," a rutin-rich drink I use for preventing varicose veins. Maybe I can get Peg to sample it, too.

Caution: Contraindications, Interactions, and Side Effects

In clinical studies, the most common side effects of butcher's broom were dizziness, dyspepsia, headache, nausea, and pruritis—no different than the placebo. Adverse effects were reported in only 0.6 percent of 5,000 patients, according to Philippe O. Szapary, M.D., and Michael D. Cirigliano, M.D.

jump-ups. In my experience, they're perfectly safe to eat; I have sampled them all. Just be sure you know what you're picking.

Witch hazel. Sold over-the-counter for treatment of hemorrhoids, witch hazel has antiseptic and astringent properties that may ease symptoms. Try using it topically, along with your standardized horse chestnut capsules or tincture.

 ## ALL IN THE FAMILY: BUCKWHEAT

Buckwheat is not, strictly speaking, a relative of horse chestnut. But I've included it here because it is one of the best sources of those capillary-strengthening compounds, rutins. Many Americans are only familiar with buckwheat as a pancake ingredient, whose flour is readily available in health food and grocery stores. But buckwheat is more than a tasty batter.

What Buckwheat Is and What It Can Do

This native of Asia and northern and southern Europe resembles a morning glory, with triangular leaves. It grows in a clambering fashion and puts forth clusters of smaller, attractive, greenish-white flowers.

In Canada, it is cultivated and used as a crop for flour. There, and in the United States, it also has been grown for soil conservation. One friend of mine is growing buckwheat sprouts, which have a nice, almost citruslike twang, he says.

Stephen Facciola, author of *Cornucopia—A Source Book of Edible Plants*, says hulled kernels or groats are used in breakfast cereals, kasha, and polenta. Buckwheat flour is made into breads and used as a thickener for gravies. Seedlings, called buckwheat lettuce, are eaten in salads and available in health food stores. A beer may be brewed from the grain and distilled into fine liquor. The seed, sprouts, and leaves are all edible, Facciola says.

In Japan, buckwheat flour is used widely as a noodle, says Tyozaburo Tanaka, Ph.D., author of *Cyclopedia of Edible Plants of the World*. If I suffered from edema or chronic venous insufficiency (CVI), I probably would add buckwheat to my herbal cabinet and use it with my horse chestnut and butcher's broom. I may just do that anyway, for triple protection. Or maybe I'll whip up a rutin-rich buckwheat cake, smothered with buckwheat flowers and sprouts and decorated with blue violets and pansies.

Caution: Contraindications, Interactions, and Side Effects

When I was a boy in North Carolina, mothers warned against carrying or eating the dangerously poisonous horse chestnut. In my *CRC Handbook of Medicinal Plants* from 1985, I even listed symptoms of toxicity: "nervous twitching of muscles, weakness, lack of coordination, dilated pupils, vomiting, diarrhea, depression, paralysis, and stupor."

How Buckwheat Can Help

Buckwheat's medicinal value has been better appreciated in Europe, where it is used for the treatment of varicose veins, CVI, and hemorrhoids. Extracts are used orally and topically.

Buckwheat also is sold as a tea. In one clinical trial, 77 patients with chronic venous insufficiency and edema were asked to drink three cups daily of a standardized buckwheat tea or one containing a placebo, according to a 1996 report in the *Quarterly Review of Natural Medicine*. After 12 weeks, the patients reported no adverse effects. But those who drank the buckwheat tea experienced significant reduction in leg volume, compared to patients who received a placebo.

Buckwheat is one of hundreds of food pharmaceuticals and thousands of medicinal plants not reviewed by Commission E. That doesn't mean it's toxic, however, or ineffective. Because it is a food, it simply doesn't require approval in Germany.

Caution: Contraindications, Interactions, and Side Effects

The *PDR for Herbal Medicines*, published in 1998 by Medical Economics, reports that there are no recorded risks or side effects when buckwheat is properly used—but large quantities are said to cause phototoxicity in grazing animals. To me, the fact that buckwheat is a food makes it safer than even standardized horse chestnut or butcher's broom, although I don't know that it's as effective.

Allergy alert. The wife of one of my chemist friends almost died after eating noodles made from buckwheat flour in Japan. She had an allergic reaction. Some people can have anaphylactic reactions to buckwheat, but this isn't common.

Rutinade

I have my own rutin-rich formula that I whip into a drink for prevention of vascular spiders and varicose veins. You might have trouble finding all of these ingredients, but you can use just a few and adjust it to your tastes. Don't use any ingredients to which you might be allergic. My "rutinade" typically contains violet flowers, eucalyptus, citrus and mulberry leaves, rhubarb, and sheep sorrel. Put about a handful of each into the blender and cover with water, a bit of sugar, and lemon to taste. Blend.

In season, violets or pansies account for a greater percentage of the ingredients. My beverages are never the same, so you should feel free to improvise, too.

Drs. Szapary and Cirigliano say a compound called aesculin, in the seeds, is largely responsible for toxicity in unprocessed horse chestnut. And of course, any medicine taken in large enough quantities can be poisonous. While the unprocessed nut is toxic, standardized capsules and tinctures are widely used as medicines. I am not afraid to take them.

Health conditions. Some sources warn not to use horse chestnut if you are pregnant or breastfeeding; are suffering from renal or hepatic insufficiency, or acute or chronic deep-vein thrombosis; or are on coumadin.

Pharmaceutical alert. I've not heard of any adverse interactions between horse chestnut and other medicinal plants or synthetic drugs.

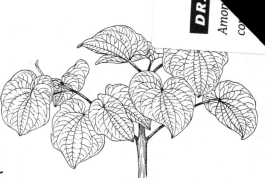

chapter eleven

Kava Kava

| LATIN NAME: *Piper methysticum* |
| FAMILY NAME: Piperaceae |

HOW COULD OUR SOCIETY have erred in readily accepting a good-morning jolt from a cup of java without ever discovering the winding-down pleasure at day's end with a cup of kava? The two beautifully balance and complement each other—one to wake up, one to wind down.

I'm a heavy coffee drinker, and while I don't often have a problem slipping off to sleep, if a touch of insomnia does come on, I wouldn't hesitate to take some kava. Usually, though, I reach for it when I want to mellow out with friends during a social occasion or, at the opposite extreme, following a stressful event. During a recent journey to the Amazon, for example, I was glad I had some handy. Whatever could go wrong did go wrong: Peruvian gardens reachable only by canoes and hour-long walks in the forest; a veritable mutiny among cranky passengers; people collapsing from severe dehydration; my sudden promotion to ticket dispenser for the entire tourist group; and the near loss of a wallet that contained my credit cards, a passport copy, and the money I set aside to buy a Peruvian guitar. It was a kava week.

Fortunately, kava and I are old friends. If everyone else knew what I know about this ancient shrub, we as a society would feel

*g Polynesians, kava is
sidered better and more so-
cially acceptable than alcohol.
That's why it's offered to the
most honored of guests.
Lyndon Johnson and Lady Bird
enjoyed it on state visits to
Pacific Island nations, and so
did Pope John Paul II. Hillary
Rodham Clinton drank some
kava during a campaign tour
of Hawaii, and the Queen of
Great Britain enjoyed "high
kava" (as opposed to "high
tea") when she stopped in Fiji
for an official state visit.*

much more at ease about our lot in the world, and fewer of us would know the dangers of addiction to Valium and other forms of pharmaceutical sedation.

What Kava Is and What It Can Do

Science has solidly established kava's ability to relax muscles and hush harried nerves. No single substance in the plant deserves sole credit. Responsibility rests with a group of chemicals called kavalactones. Found in different concentrations in different parts of the plant, each kavalactone exerts a somewhat different physiological effect. Based on what I know about how phytochemicals interact synergistically, I'd say that the kavalactones are more therapeutic in concert than if soloing separately. In other words, to bring up again a favorite refrain, there's no single magic bullet. You need the whole herbal shotgun blast.

The Kava Calm

One tremendous hurdle along the path toward establishing the superiority of herbal medicine is the dearth of research directly comparing the performance of a given plant potion to its pharmaceutical rivals. Happily, kava is an exception. Unhappily, few Americans have gotten the word. The bulk of the research has been conducted in Europe, leaving U.S. scientists, convinced that their chemistry can outsmart Mother Nature, to lag way behind. Here's what they—and you—have missed out on.

To reduce tension, stress, and anxiety, kava extract clearly and cleanly wins out over the prescription drugs with which it has been compared. It's similarly effective as tranquilizers, anxiolytics (anxiety-

If people have been doing something since time immemorial, odds are that they have a pretty good reason. As far as ingesting kava is concerned, they sure do. We now understand chemically why the plant has acquired such a long-lasting loyal following.

I hate to isolate individual compounds in a plant. They cohabitate for a reason and usually serve us best when working together, not on their own. Among the more important medicinal ingredients in kava, for instance, are substances called kavalactones. Each of them—kawain, dihydrokawain, methysticin, yangonin, desmethoxyyangonin, and dihydromethysticin—possesses slightly different physiological effects, but when they work synergistically, they're anywhere from 2 to 20 times more active.

With that in mind, I'll note that dihydrokawain (DHK) and dihydromethysticin (DHM) appear to be the most effective general relaxants and muscle relaxants of the phytochemical bunch. Together, they pack the analgesic punch of a typical 200-milligram aspirin. DHK is the primary sedative, while kawain is more of a tranquilizer. DHM gently depresses the central nervous system, as does kawain, to a lesser extent. For the most part, these phytochemicals affect only the lower central nervous system, which means they leave higher functions intact. In other words, your body mellows out, but your mind remains sharp.

In low doses, the overall kavalactonic impact is much like that of Valium or the other benzodiazepines, although it works in a manner different from this pharmaceutical family. The primary difference, a couple of studies show, is one of safety. Although physiologically similar to the benzodiazepines, kava is clearly safer, one study concluded. The plant displays no addictive potential and threatens no mental impairment. In fact, for study participants taking kava, cognitive function actually improved!

reducing agents), and other such medications, yet free of the side effects so typical of these drugs.

In one head-to-head matchup, the herbal extract was compared against two benzodiazepine tranquilizers, bromazepam and oxazepam, on 172 people with anxiety. After six weeks, researchers concluded that the natural medicine and the synthetic drug were therapeutically similar—but that kava was the obvious safer choice. It neither impairs mental reaction nor shows a potential for addiction. In fact, aside from an upset stomach or two, the only "side effect" was that the study participants' mental functions improved! Though calm of body, they remained keen of mind.

Another study, this one eight weeks long, also concluded that kava extract was comparable to and safer than benzodiazepines. Two earlier experiments reached similar conclusions about taking the shrub for anxiety, tension, and menopause-related psychosomatic complaints. A 1996 German study of 43 women and 15 men suffering from anxiety reached the same judgment.

Kava's effectiveness and safety persist even after long-term use, according to a six-month study conducted by researchers at Jena University in Germany. The trial's 101 participants had been diagnosed with anxiety that stemmed from a variety of nonpsychotic causes, including agoraphobia and other specific phobias. Half the group took 90 to 110 milligrams of a standardized kava extract containing 70 milligrams of kavalactones; the other half took placebo pills. No one, not even the researchers, knew who was taking what. In the end, the kava users' anxiety levels, unlike those who took the fake pills, improved significantly. They felt less agitated, experienced no detrimental side effects, and suffered no withdrawal problems at the end of the experiment.

Yet again, the natural medicinal compared more than favorably with Valium and its benzodiazepine brethren, especially because of the safety factor. Few studies, the researchers pointed out, have examined the long-term implications of such drugs.

I could go on, but you get the idea. As a stress buster and anxiety antidote, kava deserves a hearty "Brava! Brava!"

How Kava Can Help

Something that puts the slack back into a day's worth of high-strung nerves certainly earns a place at home at night—or whenever else you might benefit from relaxed muscles, eased pain, and somewhat numbed nerves. Insomnia is an obvious application, but pay attention: I think you'll be surprised by some of kava's other potential uses.

Depression. According to folklore, kava can be useful for mild cases of depression. Maybe. I don't think the evidence is strong. In a report issued not long ago by the federal Agency for Health Care Policy and Research, kava earned one passing reference: The report noted that no depression-related research data existed for it or another medicinal plant, valerian.

Well, perhaps the reason is that kava is more typically associated with anxiety and stress (and valerian with insomnia). Why would anyone bother to investigate a secondary use with no strong foundation? The main therapeutic plant for depression, of course, is St. John's wort, covered in chapter 13.

Genitourinary concerns. For some reason, kava takes a notable liking to the urinary tract. Its analgesic, anti-inflammatory, muscle-relaxing qualities bring relief to a range of urinary problems, particularly in women. Kavalactones also are recognized specifically for their ability to relax the uterus, which is why the shrub has been a time-honored treatment for menstrual cramps and dysmenorrhea.

For almost any achy, inflammatory urinary disorder, medical folklore includes kava in the remedy. It's been used against bladder inflammation, urethral inflammation, vaginitis, gonorrhea, cystitis, pyelitis, and burning or pain upon going to the bathroom. And while the plant is a strong diuretic, which helps encourage urination, it also supposedly helps to treat incontinence.

 HERB LORE AND MORE

In the Pacific Ocean islands of Polynesia, kava enjoys a special status that is ages old. Islanders from Hawaii and other southern Pacific nations relax by chewing on the deep-green, spadelike leaves of the cultivated plant. They also brew the plant's rhizome into a strong beverage that's drunk during religious ceremonies, special celebrations, and social rites.

Any way you cut it, the intent remains essentially the same—to relax body and mind, ease pain, and hasten sleep. Practitioners of folk medicine have prescribed it against gout, convulsions, depression, fatigue, muscle spasms, bronchitis, rheumatism, headaches, and a range of urinary problems. They've also sought its therapeutic help as a diuretic and a general tonic.

Headaches. Muscle relaxation might be the key here, but then you don't need to single out a specific reason when the herb also blunts pain, discourages muscle spasms, settles seething nerves, and cools inflammation. Two specific kavalactones, dihydrokawain and dihydromethysticin, together have the analgesic power of a 200-milligram aspirin tablet.

Hyperactivity. Drug treatment for attention deficit/hyperactivity disorder (ADHD) has been pummeled in recent years because it's given rise to a generation of school-age children who, under the dutiful advice of their doctors, pop prescription pills like candy, notably Ritalin. As I review this very sentence, the local TV news is running a rather disparaging commentary on how children as young as two are becoming hooked on these chemicals. Even the federal Drug Enforcement Administration (DEA) has warned that taking Ritalin leads to drug addiction. The DEA's concerns, though, aren't shared by the esteemed *The Journal of the American Medical Association.* The house organ for the American Medical Association has said, in essence, not to worry.

Ritalin is actually a stimulant, but it generally (though not always) calms down kids with ADHD. Caffeine, as odd as this sounds, also calms many ADHD children, although you will find the occasional hyperactive kid who's stimulated by a cup of coffee or a can of Coke.

And so it goes for kava. It tames most people, but every once in a while, it cranks someone up. That's what happened to my secretary's grandson. Upon taking an extract of the herb, he became even more hyper.

I mention kava to every mother I meet whose child has been diagnosed with this elusive condition. I'd rather that any hyperactive child or grandchild of mine at least try kava before acquiescing to a Ritalin prescription. At the least, kava seems better (and safer). At the most, it's a safer (and more natural) lifesaver.

Some alternative practitioners have praised pycnogenol, an antioxidant phytochemical in grape seed among other plants, as an antidote for hyperactivity. Maybe it works. But I'll bet a pound of kava that the kava kava plant contains similar polyphenols with similar activities.

Insomnia. No need for sleeping pills or nightcaps that whomp you with an 80-proof wallop. When worries and woes keep you wide awake, the plant's muscle-relaxing, pain-allaying, tranquillity-inducing influence is a botanical blessing.

Some people claim that kava-influenced sleep is dreamless; others say that the deep, restful slumber it facilitates is lush with vivid, epic-length imagery. Your mileage may vary, I suppose. I don't recall any obvious changes in my dreams. If you need help to fall asleep, you probably won't care whether you dream or not.

Mouth problems. While foraging the forests of Panama some three decades ago, the very first plant my Indian hosts introduced me to for a toothache was, like kava, from the Piper family. Time and distance don't seem to make a difference. Just a few years ago, again exploring the jungles, the premier plant that Peruvian Indians showed me also was a Piper.

I can't say that kava will deaden the throbbing drumbeat of a painful tooth. I can tell you, though, that your mouth gets numb when you chew on a fresh kava leaf. Imagine the possibilities from there. Jay Ram and Roy Skogstrom, two good friends of mine from Hawaii and two good kava growers on the big island there, suggest the plant has much potential for easing, if not treating, any number of mouth maladies, including a sore throat, sore gums, herpes cold sores—even, as my Panamanian and Peruvian friends promised, a toothache. An extract might work quite well as an ingredient in lozenges, mouthwashes, and toothpaste for sensitive teeth.

Other ailments. Research hasn't verified other traditional uses for kava—not yet, that is, but folklore often has a way of anticipating what science discovers much later on. One such use for kava might be against gout. Science already knows that the plant helps to counteract both tissue swelling and inflammation, two features of gout. It's just a matter of putting two and two together. Other folk medicine applications include relieving eye pain, neuralgia of the middle ear, duodenal ulcer pain, and bronchial or other complications ensuing from heart problems.

I can't offer any particular endorsements for such treatments, but if you have one of the conditions, you might consider taking some kava to see if it helps. I doubt that you'll do any harm, but you might do yourself some good. And whether the condition responds or not, at least you'll feel more relaxed and sleep better.

How to Take It and How Much

Though traditionalists more commonly use kava's roots, if you had your own nature's "farmacy," you could snip off a leaf or two whenever you wanted to take the edge off the day. I'm proud of my greenhouse kava plant, the one *People Weekly* photographed for its February 1, 1999 issue, and I certainly don't want to uproot it or pick it apart. Instead, I have a cache of the powdered extract that I bring out to share with special people on special occasions or even just lazy afternoons. I host my own version of a kava tea ceremony.

Supplements. For you, though, standardized supplements are the way to go. On the label, look for a statement attesting that the capsules therein contain a standardized extract that provides a specific amount of kavalactones per dosage. You don't want just a certain one; you want the whole kavalactone complex.

Percentages and milligrams will vary among manufacturers. Most of the clinical studies used an extract standardized for 70 percent kavalactones at a daily dosage of 210 milligrams. The *Protocol Journal of Botanical Medicine* suggests taking an extract standardized at 40 to 70 milligrams of kavalactones twice a day for up to four to six months, while Commission E (a German panel of experts roughly equivalent to the U.S. Food and Drug Administration) recommends 60 to 120 milligrams of kavalactones daily for no more than three months.

Tinctures and extracts. Other suggested dosages I've seen include 1 to 3 milliliters of kava tincture daily, 2 to 4 milliliters daily of a liquid root extract, or 10 to 30 drops four times a day of an alcohol extract.

Dried root. Still another recommended dosage is 1.5 to 3 grams of dried kava root.

The right dosage for you will depend on a handful of factors, including your weight, your individual body chemistry, and your sensitivity to the kavalactones. But then, the same can be said of any substance, natural or synthetic. What you can reliably count on is that the more kava you take, the more you'll feel its effects.

Another factor to consider is timing. For stress relief or muscle aches during the day, you might want to take a smaller amount. In the evening, you could try a little more, if necessary, for general relaxation. And for help with insomnia, take it an hour or so before bedtime.

Useful Combinations

If kava can't ease your weary, worried brow, nature offers hundreds of recourses that you can try alone or along with kava. None of the ones I recommend possesses the side effects or addictive potential of prescription and over-the-counter tranquilizers.

But before seeking out a particular herb, I think I'd start off by exercising a little more, walking a little more, cutting back on afternoon caffeine consumption (I always switch to decaf after a few cups of the "hard" stuff), and eating more foods that provide the essential amino acid L-tryptophan, a main nutrient for mental serenity and relaxation.

Relaxation and Insomnia

Chamomile. Like Hawaiians, who balance their morning Kona coffee with afternoon kava, Latin Americans have an end-of-day counterpart to their eye-opening brew. They call it manzanilla, but you know it as chamomile. Apigenin is one of the active ingredients in this plant, which you can drink as a very gentle tea right before turning down the covers.

Foods. All plant (and probably all animal) foods contain some amount of natural tryptophan. Among the better sources are almonds, barley, mung beans, kidney and lima beans, sesame seeds, pumpkin seeds, spinach, evening primrose seed, and watercress.

If that doesn't do it for you, try some of the other plants suggested here, either alone or in combination.

Lavender. The numerous compounds in this plant and its purple blossoms slow nerve impulses and calm the central nervous system—if, that is, you get the right species and variety. Some types, particularly Spanish lavender, exert the opposite effect. Tinctures and teas are worthwhile, but the most potent form is the essential oil, which you should use only externally. Do not ingest the oil. Instead, dilute it with almond oil and rub some on your skin, or add a little bit, along with some lemon balm, to your bath water. I predict you'll fall asleep more easily and sleep solidly. But do not sleep in the tub.

Lemon balm. You'll put a churning stomach to rest, too, if you use this plant to relax. Also called melissa, it makes a great before-bed tea. Some of its active tranquilizing compounds, known as terpenes, appear in such herbs as ginger, basil, clove, and juniper, though perhaps not in quite the right blend that gives this weed its good sleep-promoting reputation.

Passionflower. In Great Britain, several dozen over-the-counter sleep nostrums contain this natural relaxant. If you can't find a tincture, you'll have to take the whole herb (anywhere between four and eight grams). Low doses ease anxiety; higher doses work more like a sedative. Even Germany's Commission E approved it for nervous restlessness and noted its lack of side effects, interactions, and contraindications. Passionflower is native to America. Too bad it's better studied and more frequently used overseas.

Valerian. This herb stinks—quite literally. But it's probably the most powerful of the other plant options I've listed, a key ingredient in some 80 British sleep aids. If you cannot or will not acquire a taste for it as a tea, get a tincture or a supplement that contains a root ex-

---

DR. DUKE'S RECIPES

Cream of Serenity Soup

Here's a kava option or accompaniment—a suggested soup to help you sleep, or at least wind down at the end of a stressful day.

Start with mung beans, kidney beans, and/or limas—all rich in natural tryptophan, a substance which promotes serenity and relaxation. Toss in some celery and some tomato, which contains nine different sleep-inducing chemicals, then flavor the concoction with any of the spices—ginger, basil, thyme, cinnamon—that are rich in natural sedative compounds.

Truly a recipe for relaxation!

tract. Again, don't settle for an extract of just one or two of the plant's active ingredients. None is necessarily better than the others. This time-tested stress buster and sleep promoter contains more than a dozen sedative-like chemicals, and they work best synergistically, not by themselves. Always remember Duke's Dictum: The whole phytochemical potpourri is almost always better than the sum of its parts.

Oral Assistants

Kava helps deaden the pain associated with toothaches and other mouth-related woes. If you don't feel any relief, you have a couple of alternatives:

Clove. As an oil that's rubbed directly on the affected tooth, clove proves superior to all other ingredients commonly found in toothache remedies, according to a group of scientists reporting to the Food and Drug Administration (FDA). In fact, it was the only substance that effectively and safely brought temporary relief from pain.

Willow. I've occasionally chewed on a piece of willow bark to soothe a throbbing tooth. Once softened, wad up the bark and gently press it into the site of pain.

Other herbs that might help anesthetize an aching tooth include ginger, prickly ash, and the aptly named toothache tree. Or sink your teeth into a capsaicin-rich hot pepper or black pepper (the latter is related to kava). Capsaicin has an outstanding reputation for relieving pain. I've never investigated its use for a toothache, but it might take your mind off the pain for a while.

Don't forget that the relief these herbs provides is only temporary. See a dentist as soon as you can.

Cramp Control

Of the genitourinary problems that kava has been used against, dysmenorrhea responds most reliably. For stronger alleviation from monthly menstrual pain, you can combine kava with a few other herbs:

Black haw. You'd expect that something more commonly called "cramp bark" would live up to its name, and this herb certainly does. For menstrual pain, I'd recommend it as a first resort. At least four of its compounds help to relax the uterus. *Viburnum opulus*, which is right now flowering in the Green Farmacy Garden, has the same effect.

Ginger. Another reliable remedy for menstrual pain, ginger has six anticramp chemicals and at least another six pain-assuaging substances. It has a long history as a dysmenorrhea treatment and a worldwide reputation for helping to induce menstruation.

So reliable is the latter effect that pregnant women might wish to avoid taking ginger, although my guess is that it would take a lot more than the normal medicinal dose to cause any problems.

Raspberry. We're not sure what the active ingredients are, but raspberry leaf tea has racked up a nice record for soothing menstrual cramps. It works well against pregnancy-related uterine discomfort, too, according to women herbal experts. Blackberry, boysenberry, and wineberry, I suspect, could serve as similarly effective substitutes.

Caution: Contraindications, Interactions, and Side Effects

If you brewed up a big, big batch of kava and drank roughly 13 liters a day, your skin eventually could turn scaly and yellow, your eyes might get red, and some hair might fall out. You also might lose a little muscle coordination and have some difficulty breathing.

I trust that no one capable of reading this book is foolish enough to consume such a large amount, which is about 100 times greater than the typical therapeutic dose. I do, however, appreciate inquisitive scientists' concern about the impact of such profligacy, wildly unrealistic as it might be.

Beware the Bum Rap

Even when used in far more rational ways, kava has been the victim of a bum rap. Excessive consumption is alleged to be intoxicating, and some of our supposed guardians of public health have gone as far as to classify the shrub as a narcotic and a hypnotic. Perhaps they're confusing drunkenness with relaxation or have put too much stock in Polynesian lore. They need to calm down.

In truth, kavalactones are not hallucinogenic, nor do they act like a narcotic. They are definitely not addictive, and they most certainly do not create a dependency. I have no reason to believe that kava is any more addictive than any other pleasurable substance. Without a doubt, it's far less addictive than tobacco and alcohol. And in medicinal dosages, it does not impair your mental faculties, as alcohol does. It's probably less habit-forming than coffee.

By any stretch of the definition, I have never felt "intoxicated" after ingesting kava, whatever its form. I doubt that you will, either, if you take it in proper medicinal dosages. At the same time, I readily acknowledge that some "kava cults" are out there for the mood-altering ride rather than the health benefits, and overindulgence does present concerns, as does overindulgence of any substance, legal or not, regulated or not. Drink 13 liters of water a day and you might experience untoward side effects, too.

Legitimate Cautions

What, then, are the realistic concerns? Not many. For the most part, with sane, rational use, you have a slim, very tiny chance of getting a headache or a stomachache. Or you might feel dizzy. With continued regular use, and certainly with chronic abuse, your skin could turn a slight shade of yellow, a condition, called "kawism" or kava dermatitis, that reverses itself once you stop ingesting so much. I wouldn't worry unnecessarily. As I mentioned, you shouldn't ingest the plant on a daily basis for several months in a row.

Kava doesn't mix well with everything. Here are several points to keep in mind:

Drugs. Barbiturates, tranquilizers, antidepressants, and central nervous system depressants probably don't interact well. The drugs and the plant might enhance one another's actions, and you could end up overmedicated.

Doctors and pharmacists, I'll guess, would tell you to lay off the herbs. I, on the other hand, would probably go in the opposite direction: If you can, lay off the synthetic medications. Recruit the help of a holistic physician, if need be. Synthetics, in my opinion, are more likely to have detrimental side effects than the natural medicines with which we've co-evolved for millions of years.

Alcohol. As with pharmaceuticals, the effects could be additive. So it may not be a good idea to chase down your daily dose of kava with an alcoholic beverage.

I feel obligated to issue that warning, because everyone reacts differently to different substances. At the same time, I feel compelled to tell you what I'm about to do. As I write this, it's late. I've spent the last 12 hours proofreading chapters for this book. You might think I'd be dead-tired and ready for bed, but I'm actually tense from such stressful work. Thinking about this plant and what it does has just given me an idea for a new nightcap: a vodka tincture of kava with lemon balm and lavender. I'll dub it the Kava Kooler. Just pondering the ingredients allays my frayed nerves. While conservatism prevents me from recommending it to anyone else, I'll wager that I sleep better after my Kava Kooler.

Pregnancy. Here's another cover-the-fanny caveat dictated by conservatism and litigiousness: Women who are pregnant or breast-feeding a newborn shouldn't use the plant at all. There is no indication at all, mind you, that kava poses a threat in this regard. In the absence of proof of safety, though, conservative medical authorities always cop out and assume that an herbal medicine might imperil pregnant women, breastfeeding mothers, babies, and children.

I can't say otherwise, because I'm not a physician or a medical expert. What I can tell you is that pharmaceutical firms have not done much pediatric-related safety research on their drugs. For a majority of the medications out there, studies attesting to their safety for pregnant or nursing women or children simply do not exist.

Libido. Don't expect kava to put you in the mood for anything other than relaxation—especially if you have amour in mind. While making you feel mellow and mushy, the plant tends to lower your interest in sexual activities.

Again, this comes from anecdotal reports I've culled from the literature. I have no verification, from personal experience or personal contacts, that kava saps your sex drive. You might very well find that kava enhances love-making. But some reports to the contrary make me duty-bound to say that if you take some before going to bed, make sure all you plan to do is sleep.

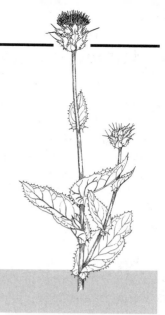

chapter twelve

Milk Thistle

LATIN NAME: *Silybum marianum*
FAMILY NAME: Asteraceae

I TAKE MILK THISTLE to prevent or slow the deterioration of the liver, that overworked organ that detoxifies the blood. Although better known in Europe than here in the United States, "milk thistle can't be beat as a liver protector," says Varro E. Tyler, Ph.D., Sc.D., professor emeritus of pharmacognosy at Purdue University and co-author of *Tyler's Honest Herbal*. I agree. And there are times when I need the best of liver protectors.

When the Christmas holiday approaches, I'm much more likely to take some of the herbs in my geriatric dozen. With all the traditional traveling, visiting, and feasting, there's bound to be more bending of the elbow. That's when I rely on the biblical milk thistle.

And when I'm on the road any time of year, I always take milk thistle capsules with me. This herb can protect my liver from pollution in the airplane, at the airport, on the road to the hotel, and in the hotel itself (the toxic building syndrome is no myth). In the hotel bar, of course, there is more travel-related wining and dining to protect against, too.

I get a lot of mail from people who tell me that milk thistle really helped them with serious health problems. I really think it is one of the most effective herbs.

HERB LORE AND MORE

In folklore, there are references to the white marks on milk thistle leaves as splashes of the Virgin Mary's milk. And in fact, this herb has a traditional use of helping mothers produce milk to breastfeed their babies.

The January 1997 *Review of Natural Products*, a respected newsletter, pointed out that milk thistle has been used for liver problems for over 2,000 years, and that's why it is still my liver-protecting herb of choice. In ancient Rome, Pliny suggested that it carries off bile. Premier English herbalist Culpepper suggested it was good for jaundice and for removing liver obstructions. (They were right!)

The liver "purifies" the blood, and that's why the herbalists of old considered all the liver tonics to be blood purifiers, sometimes using the archaic word (at least in my vocabulary) depurative. My *Dorland's Illustrated Medical Dictionary* defines *depurative* as "tending to purify or cleanse." I can't quibble about the depurativity of the milk thistle.

Milk thistle also has a history of use as an alterative (something that helps the body return to its normal state), laxative, purgative, and stimulant. It has been traditionally used to purge bile, soothe mucous membranes, regulate menses, expel phlegm, stop the flow of blood, and promote sweating.

Milk thistle has also been mentioned as a folkloric remedy for anthrax, asthma, bladder stones, cancer, catarrh, chest ailments, dropsy, fever, bleeding from the lungs or bronchia, hepatitis, rabies, jaundice, vaginal discharge, malaria, melancholy, piles, plague, pleurisy, spasms, and spleen and uterus problems.

In the Middle East, a flower infusion is used as an alterative, a cooling remedy, and a tonic. Boiled in vinegar, the leaves are used for skin ailments and tonics. The astringent root is used for hemorrhoids and worms. The Lebanese also used the seed infusion for stones of the gallbladder and liver, to promote the flow of milk, and as a stimulant and tonic.

Albrecht von Haller, Swiss anatomist, surgeon, and botanist, suggested milk thistle for liver ailments back in 1755.

What Milk Thistle Is and What It Can Do

Milk thistle is native to the warm, dry areas of southern Europe and northern Africa. It is a beautiful, sturdy plant with shiny, spiny, mottled foliage. My milk thistle plants have a very attractive pattern of white veins two to three millimeters wide separated by light green interspaces. The flowers are fuzzy, soft, and purplish.

Incredibly Edible

All parts of the milk thistle are said to be edible, and this plant has long been used for food in the countries surrounding the Mediterranean. Young leaves can be trimmed of prickles and added to salads or steamed for a vegetable. They taste a little bitter and astringent and sort of get gummy as you chew.

The roots can be prepared and cooked like salsify or eaten raw. The young flower buds can be steamed and eaten like those of the globe artichoke, a close relative. (In fact, just this morning I picked and ate some buds from a six-foot plant.)

Like many members of the daisy family, the scorched roots and seeds of milk thistle have been used as a coffee substitute, the seed cake is used for cattle fodder, and the seed oil for food or lubrication.

I have enjoyed munching the seeds like sunflower seeds and can see a great potential for the seeds as beer nuts to serve in bars where the drinkers are worried about their livers but don't have enough sense to taper off. Birds like the seeds, too.

Milk thistle is not on the Food and Drug Administration's (FDA's) "generally recognized as safe" (GRAS) list, but it is what I call "generally recognized as food" (GRAF). In my subjective scoring, milk thistle rates safer than coffee. To remind the FDA that milk thistle is a food, perhaps we should call it the "milk artichoke."

Traditionally, a tea made from various parts of the plant has been used to improve the appetite, alleviate indigestion, and as a liver tonic. And true to its name, milk thistle also has a long folk history of helping nursing mothers increase milk secretion.

Only recently, however, has science begun to investigate the chemistry and physiologic effects of this plant. Commercial preparations of

The fatty acid composition of the oil produced from milk thistle seeds is similar to sunflower seed oil and can be substituted in some pharmaceutical and cosmetic formulations.

the seed extracts are manufactured in Europe and are currently used to treat jaundice, cirrhosis, hepatitis, and liver poisoning from chemicals or from drug and alcohol abuse.

If you are the gardening type, you can buy milk thistle seeds from an herb catalog and grow the plants, but I wouldn't advise trying to harvest the seeds yourself. This thistle's spines can be a real challenge, even if you arm yourself with long gloves and pruners.

I must also caution that milk thistle can be invasive. It's becoming a weed here in my Green Farmacy Garden where it is refusing to stay in its four assigned plots: aging and senescence, alcohol and addictions, hepatitis and liver problems, and ulcers. It is a very attractive weed, however.

How Milk Thistle Can Help

In reviewing the literature on herbs that protect the liver, I concluded that silymarin from the milk thistle, *Silybum marianum*, seems to be the most promising natural compound both for preventing damage to the liver and for correcting a damaged liver. And even if you have a healthy liver, milk thistle can help it remove toxins more effectively.

Meet Your Liver

Few vital organs are so vital as the liver. About the same color and size as a football, the liver is your body's chemical factory.

It produces important proteins for blood plasma. These include albumin, which regulates the exchange of water between blood and tissues; complement, a group of proteins crucial to the immune system; coagulation factors; and globin for hemoglobin, which carries oxygen in the blood. The liver also produces cholesterol.

With the recent surge of interest in alternative therapies in the United States, doctors began to notice that more and more of their patients were taking the herb milk thistle. To find out why, a group of researchers in the Gastroenterology Division of Oregon Health Sciences University in Portland conducted a study of milk thistle's history, pharmacology, and properties. They also looked at clinical trials pertaining to patients with acute and chronic liver disease. They found indications that silymarin, milk thistle's main active compound, is an antioxidant that protects cells and inhibits the growth of tumors. They also found studies to suggest that silymarin protects and promotes the regeneration of liver cells.

In another instance of Europe being more herbally advanced, Commission E, the German government's expert panel that judges the safety and effectiveness of medicinal herbs, has already approved milk thistle seeds or seed extracts as supportive treatment for cirrhosis and chronic inflammatory liver conditions such as hepatitis.

In the 1960s, German scientists identified a group of active ingredients in milk thistle, found mainly in its seeds, which collectively is called silymarin. The four main, closely related compounds are isosilybinin, silychristin, silydianin, and silybinin. The later accounts for about 50 percent of a plant's silymarin.

Silymarin protects the liver in two ways. It strengthens the outer membranes of liver cells, which prevents toxins from penetrating. It also stimulates an enzymatic action that in turn increases protein synthesis, which stimulates the ability of the liver to form new cells and repair itself.

The silybinin component of silymarin has been shown to reduce cholesterol in bile. And because silymarin increases bile solubility, it can help prevent or alleviate gallstones.

Many European studies have investigated the effects of silymarin on liver diseases. One Finnish study showed a significant decrease of elevated enzymes after patients took milk thistle capsules. More recently, an Italian study showed that as an antioxidant, silymarin reduced damage to liver cells caused by chronic use of some prescription drugs.

After a meal, the liver converts amino acids to glucose, proteins, or urea, which is excreted by the kidneys in the urine. The liver's bile also enables better digestion of the fats (some of them toxic) you may have consumed.

The liver is also your blood's filtration system. It extracts drugs and poisons, such as alcohol or pollutants, alters their chemical structure, and excretes them in the bile. If the filter doesn't work properly, dangerous toxins may remain in the body.

Here's what milk thistle can do to help.

Alcoholism. There are an estimated 11 million alcoholics in the United States, with 200,000 dying from the disease every year. In urban areas, alcoholic liver disease is the fourth leading cause of death in 25- to 64-year-old men. Chronic consumption of alcohol increases enzyme activities in the liver, which leads to malnutrition and ethanol toxicity as well as an increase in ethanol-induced free radicals.

As an antioxidant and a cell protector, the silymarin in milk thistle can protect the liver from chemical damage, including ethanolic damage, and that's the main reason I'm taking it.

Cirrhosis. Alcohol abuse or viral hepatitis can damage the healthy cells of the liver and replace them with scar tissue. The result is a group of serious, chronic, degenerative diseases called cirrhosis. The impaired liver cannot carry out its many important functions, such as storing and filtering blood or producing bile. Even liver cancer may ensue.

Researchers at the University of Vienna in Austria studied the effects of silymarin on patients with cirrhosis of the liver due to alcohol. They found that patients who took milk thistle extract lived significantly longer, with no negative side effects.

Hepatitis. An inflammation of the liver, there are various types of hepatitis. Most are caused by viral infection, but hepatitis may also be caused by an overdose of drugs, such as acetaminophen, the active ingredient in Tylenol. Exposure to certain chemicals, such as dry cleaning agents, or alcohol abuse may result in hepatitis.

Inflammation damages liver cells, and the most severe cases may result in liver failure and death. Hepatitis caused by heavy drinking may result in the cell destruction and scarring that leads to liver cirrhosis.

Infection can be flu-like, with nausea and vomiting. Jaundice, a yellowish hue to the skin, is the most noticeable symptom of hepatitis, but symptoms can be less apparent. Chronic hepatitis may be marked by nothing more than a vague feeling of being unwell.

With its ability to protect and regenerate injured liver cells, milk thistle has been used successfully to treat hepatitis.

I recently heard from a colleague whose sister had been diagnosed with infectious hepatitis. "You could only describe her skin and eye color as 'sunflower yellow'!" she wrote. "Tests showed her liver was functioning at 40 percent. She had a vitamin K shot and started taking milk thistle tablets. When she had a second liver function test three weeks later, it showed the liver functioning at 82 percent! The doctor says it was unbelievable.

He told her that recovery time from hepatitis is up to nine months!"

Pollution. In my travels I meet a lot of pollutants more dangerous and less relaxing than alcohol. Milk thistle, in the same way that it protects the liver from alcoholic intoxication, can help prevent damage caused by environmental toxins. Its active ingredient, silymarin, helps strengthen cell membranes to prevent toxic substances from entering liver cells.

German studies have shown that giving rats silymarin beforehand protected them from the effects of pollutants such as carbon tetrachloride, which is sometimes concentrated by industrial use.

(continued on page 194)

WHAT NEW RESEARCH TELLS US

Recent research is uncovering some exciting possibilities for milk thistle.

Help for Hepatitis C

Hepatitis C is caused by a virus identified in the late 1980s. It is spread in ways similar to the HIV infection. Scientists call it the "silent epidemic" because its symptoms of fatigue and nausea may not appear for decades. Some estimates put the number of infected Americans at more than 4 million.

The usual treatment for hepatitis C is interferon, a generic antiviral (and anticancer) drug. Injections of interferon are expensive, have a low success rate, and can cause serious side effects. Here's definitely a case where I'd prefer the herbal alternative. I've had some encouraging reports from therapists who have used milk thistle to treat patients with hepatitis C.

My friend Steven Morris, N.D., a naturopathic physician in Seattle, put a patient with hepatitis C on an alcohol-free, liver-cleansing diet and taught him stress management techniques. He also prescribed some daily herbs, including 150 milligrams of *Silybum marianum*. After three months, the patient's liver enzymes returned to normal limits, and the signs and symptoms of the disease improved.

Amanda McQuade Crawford, a British-trained phytotherapist, founding member of the American Herbalists Guild, and founder and director of the National College of Phytotherapy in New Mexico, added silymarin and dandelion to the treatment of one of her hepatitis C patients. She also added a strong diuretic (Lasix) to the usual interferon, an antiviral drug. In three months, her patient no longer needed the Lasix and tests showed improved liver enzymes and viral load. It may be an instance of a gentle diuretic and a gentle antiviral improving the effectiveness and minimizing the side effects of a strong antiviral and a strong diuretic.

Crawford cautions that people with hepatitis C respond differently to herbs, drugs, and nutrition, and is hesitant to prescribe any single natural or alternative approach. "Complex humans with equally complex health conditions take a little more than substituting an herb for a prescription," she warns.

Treatment for Mushroom Poisoning

Each year, thousands of people become ill, and a few even die, from eating poisonous mushrooms. Most of these are children, who don't yet know there are good mushrooms and bad mushrooms. Often the victims of mushroom poisonings are immigrants, who mistake poisonous fungi for edible look-alikes that grow in their native countries. Sometimes it is the so-called mushroom experts who make a mistake.

The most serious cases of mushroom poisoning, and more than 90 percent of the deaths, are traced to the death cap mushroom, *Amanita phalloides*. This species, as well as several others in its genus, contain deadly amatoxin poisons that are not destroyed by heat, water, or drying.

These toxins can kill liver cells. The first signs of amanita poisoning are vomiting, cramping, and diarrhea, followed by liver damage, and in the most serious cases, kidney damage and liver failure. Sometimes the only recourse is a liver transplant—unless you live in Europe.

While milk thistle is not widely used in the United States, European research suggests that silybinin, one of the compounds in silymarin, a flavonoid component of milk thistle seed, can be used to treat severe amanita mushroom poisoning. In one experiment, every animal given silymarin and/or silybinin treatment before being poisoned with mushrooms survived. And when silybinin was given intravenously to humans who accidentally ate death cap mushrooms, the death rate was dramatically reduced.

In 1996, a Netherlands medical journal told of a husband and wife who ate *Amanita phalloides* mushrooms and developed symptoms of poisoning 18 hours later. When their livers and kidneys began to deteriorate, they were treated intravenously with silybinin, penicillin, and glucose. After three days, organ failure was reversed. Researchers noted that both silybinin and penicillin prevent amatoxin uptake into liver cells, but also noted that the penicillin treatment can have serious side effects if used for more than three days.

How to Take It and How Much

Silymarin, milk thistle's active ingredient, is concentrated from milk thistle seeds and sold in standardized capsule form or extracts. The capsules I take are standardized at 80 percent silymarin. The recommended average daily dose is 200 to 400 milligrams of silymarin, but I don't take it regularly unless I'm traveling or celebrating.

Some herbalists say that it's better to eat the seeds or capsules than make a tea or infusion of the seeds. Silymarin is barely soluble in water and poorly absorbed from the stomach, so it needs to be concentrated and standardized for oral use.

I've never been desperate enough to harvest milk thistle seeds myself, but if I were, I'd get out the scissors and a pair of long, tough

 ## ALL IN THE FAMILY: ARTICHOKE

Another milk thistle relative, the artichoke is native to the Mediterranean, and it's now widely grown along parts of the U.S. west coast. I'll eat artichokes when I'm in California and they are served up for me. You can find them in almost any supermarket produce section anywhere in the United States, however.

What Artichoke Is and What It Can Do

The artichoke (technically, the globe artichoke as opposed to the rootcrop called Jerusalem artichoke, another good inulin source) is a thistlelike plant grown for its edible flower buds. Globe artichoke flowers are very similar to those of the milk thistle, although globe artichokes do not have all those dangerous spiny bristles. Jerusalem artichokes, on the other hand, more closely resemble a yellow echinacea. The Japanese name for the artichoke, chosen azami, means "Korean thistle."

Diabetes. Artichoke flower heads are reported to be a source of inulin for diabetics.

Liver protection. Artichokes seem to share many flavonoids and lignans that may account for the liver-protective properties of milk thistle.

Rheumatism and dropsy. Artichoke leaves have been used as a diuretic for treating rheumatism and dropsy.

gloves. Eating the seeds can be effective, because all sorts of things happen in the stomach that don't happen in water or alcohol extracts. I'd estimate you'd have to eat about half an ounce of seeds to get the equivalent of an average daily dose of silymarin.

Useful Combinations

Taking silymarin with other food-grade herbs in the same family that have a nice liver protective reputation makes good sense.

Dandelion. Dandelion is one such "family" plant. The flowers of dandelion are very rich in lecithin, a liver protector. In another case of

What New Research Tells Us

A few recent European studies have looked at the ability of artichoke extracts to promote health. One termed it useful for bile secretion dysfunction. Another study found that artichokes are rich in luteolin, a protective antioxidant.

In yet another study, German laboratory experiments looked at how artichoke extracts affected rat liver cells in the test tube. The extract's antioxidant properties protected the liver cells from damage, and also inhibited the formation of cholesterol.

How to Take It and How Much

Artichoke supplements can be found in capsule form, but eating them as a sweet, mild vegetable is to me a much more pleasurable way to benefit from its healthful properties.

Caution

Some people may be sensitive to artichokes and may develop a rash or other skin irritation after touching them. Christopher Hobbs, herbalist, botanist, and author, suggests you stay away from artichokes if you have ulcerative colitis, gallstones, or allergies. But I'll continue to enjoy them as a vehicle for rich, delicious sauces or melted butter.

science trying to imitate nature, a new Italian drug combines the antioxidant silybinin with lecithin. Other beneficial plants in the milk thistle family include burdock and artichoke.

Echinacea. If I had hepatitis C, I'd be taking the floral extracts of echinacea (see chapter 5) along with my milk thistle and heavy-duty

 # ALL IN THE FAMILY: BURDOCK

The milk thistle hails from one of the largest plant families, the *Asteraceae*, formerly known as the *Compositae*. This family includes everything from lettuce to sunflowers, but there are a couple relatives that share many chemicals and activities with milk thistle. One of them is burdock. To most Americans, burdock is a big, bad weed, but lots of bad weeds can be good plants.

What Burdock Is and What It Can Do

Burdock can grow up to six feet tall. One way to identify burdock is by the flowers. Burdock has pink, thistlelike flowers that attach themselves to everything, especially dogs and children. (This plant is named "burr dock" for good reason.)

Burdock is a biennial, and if you want to harvest the root, you have to dig it up in the first year. In the second year, the root gets all withered and dry as the energy moves into the flower.

Herb Lore and More

When Europeans arrived in North America, they probably brought burdock with them (likely attached to their clothes). They used it as a liver tonic and blood purifier. They also scorched its roots for a coffee substitute.

It quickly naturalized (grew like a weed) and was adopted by the native tribes, who probably learned about its uses from the newcomers. In the mid-South, the Cherokee used burdock to treat small kidney stones, rheumatism, scurvy, and "weakly females." They also used burdock root or seed infusion to cleanse the blood and for venereal disease. The Micmacs of maritime eastern Canada used burdock buds and roots for skin problems, sores, and chancres. Other tribes made poultices of the boiled leaves for sores, and the Iroquois ate dried burdock roots in winter and young burdock leaves in spring.

medications. Flowers of echinacea are the best source I've found for cichoric acid, which, through its reported anti-integrase activity, may slow reproduction of viruses. Some echinacea tablets are now standardized for cichoric acid.

Christopher Hobbs, herbalist, botanist, and author, mixes milk

How Burdock Can Help

Believe me, I would take the "food farmaceutical," burdock, if I were targeted for leukemia or lymphoma, or if I had AIDS.

Like milk thistle, burdock can help protect the liver from alcohol intoxication as well as environmental toxins. Like milk thistle, bitter burdock can stimulate the flow of digestive juices, especially bile secretion, and help the kidneys function. It's also recognized as a diuretic.

Cancer. Burdock has some anticancer activity, especially against cancers like lymphoma. A 1998 report in the *Review of Natural Products* suggests that both burdock and blessed thistle (a close milk thistle relative) contain two important substances, artcigenin and trachelogenin, that have elsewhere been shown to be active against leukemia, lymphoma, and various types of tumors.

HIV/AIDS. According to the *Review of Natural Products*, burdock juice or extracts weakened or killed HIV cells in the test tube.

How to Take It and How Much

Burdock root capsules are available from some natural products companies, but I'm happy to harvest my own and weed my garden at the same time. Capsules are an easier choice for most people, though, so go with 475 milligram capsules 3 times daily or as directed on the label.

Caution

Burdock scores higher on my safety scale than most medicinal herbs, wholesome teas, and many food plants. The Japanese call it *gobo*, and they grow it as a crop for its edible roots, believing it enhances endurance and sexual virility. Maybe it is the *gobo* rather than soybeans (or mung beans and their sprouts, green tea, wasabi, or seaweed) that contributes to their lower incidence of breast cancer.

thistle seed into his liver-digestive combo, which also includes artichoke leaf, dandelion root, turmeric rhizome, skullcap, and California coast sage.

Caution: Contraindications, Interactions, and Side Effects

Germany's Commission E (a panel of experts roughly the equivalent to the U.S. Food and Drug Administration) reports no known contraindications or drug interactions for milk thistle, the fruit. Occasional mild laxative effects have been noted, but if you stick to the recommended dose, there should be no problems.

chapter thirteen

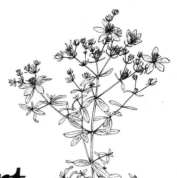

St. John's Wort

LATIN NAME: *Hypericum perforatum*
FAMILY NAME: Clusiaceae

ST. JOHN'S WORT is a happy plant. Just looking at its yellow, star-shaped flowers is enough to lift my spirits. But in the winter of 1998, I reached for this weedy perennial for more than its aesthetic qualities. Knowing the herb is a proven antidepressant as well as a potential treatment for a variety of ailments, I supplemented with St. John's wort capsules four times a day to shake my winter doldrums.

Optimistic and energetic by nature, I typically work 12-hour days at my computer, walk daily in and around my six-acre herbal vineyard, and travel the world to forage for plants or talk about them. One of my associates jokes that she hardly has the energy to keep up with me, even though her years tally far fewer than my 70.

Thankfully, I have never suffered from debilitating, down-and-out depression. But every fall, as the daylight hours wane, my mood fades too. I lose my usual enthusiasm. I feel out of sorts.

Looking back, I think I've always been less motivated in fall and winter. As a boy living in the South, where sunlight is plentiful, at least in summer, this was not a problem for me. As an adult living in Maryland, farther from the equator, my annual dose of sun is not as potent. And I sense the subtle effects.

In recent years, science has given a name to this common human experience: seasonal affective disorder, or SAD. While it is a form of depression—affecting 10 million people in the United States, the National Institute of Mental Health reports—it usually is mild and short lived. When there is less daytime, our brains don't get as much light by way of our eyes. That translates into fewer nourishing neurochemicals that fuel our sense of well-being.

Annual jaunts to Peru and other South American climes are my favorite antidote for the winter blues. But in 1998, I had no trip planned. So, instead, I took standardized hypericum capsules for the first time. After all, years of research and conversations with colleagues and friends had convinced me hypericum was not to be ignored. Now, I consider it part of my herbal arsenal, a kind of vacation in a bottle, when a trip to the Amazon is out of the question.

What St. John's Wort Is and What It Can Do

You've probably heard something about St. John's wort—or St. Joan's wort, as my herbalist friend Susun Weed, author of *Breast Cancer? Breast Health! The Wise Woman Way*, dubs it. Maybe you know of someone who claims this herb—in capsule form, tincture, or tea—has helped her ward off SAD or full-blown depression.

Hypericum's been much more popular in the United States since 1997 when a national television program aired a report on the herb's reputed antidepressant properties. The plant—and products made from it—became downright hard to find.

Now, it's available everywhere—in health food stores, pharmacies, and supermarkets and in products from well-known vitamin manufacturers. Even in potato chips. Its reputation is growing beyond that of an antidepressant. Some of the phytochemicals in St. John's wort are believed to be helpful in staving off HIV, the virus that causes AIDS, and in the topical treatment of herpes viruses and first-degree burns, cuts, and wounds. They show promise, too, in easing the pain and swelling of arthritis and fibromyalgia and the discomfort associated with menopause and perimenopause as well as other medical conditions. That's why St. John's wort is among Duke's Dozen.

This pretty perennial is native to Europe, where its use dates back 2,000 years. In their book, *Rational Therapy—A Physician's Guide to Herbal Medicine*, Volker Schulz, Rudolf Hansel, and Varro E. Tyler say it grows wild as a weed in Asia and North and South America. I find it grows in most temperate climates, especially in dry sunny locations.

Some people claim the herb gets its name from St. John's Day (June 24), when it typically blooms, although there are other explanations. Wort, incidentally, has no relation to the unsightly skin growth (spelled warts) that toads are infamous—incorrectly—for passing along. It simply is old English for "plant." In earlier times, the herb was said to expel evil spirits in those who ingested it. The Latin name, *Hypericum*, is based on the Greek word for "over an apparition."

Emotional Health

Schulz, Hansel, and Tyler suggest that Paracelsus, the sixteenth-century Swiss physician and alchemist, knew of hypericum's effectiveness in treating psychiatric conditions and that German poet-physician Justinus Kerner reported its use in mood disorders in the early nineteenth century.

In more recent years, though, the herb was pushed aside in favor of synthetic antidepressants. Then, in the late twentieth century, reports of its usefulness began to pour in once again. Most came from Germany, where the value of herbal medicines has been more readily embraced.

In 1984, Commission E (a German panel of experts roughly equivalent to the U.S. Food and Drug Administration) approved hypericum for relief of mild to moderate depression and anxiety associated with it. As study after study cited its effectiveness, St. John's wort became the leading antidepressant in Germany. There, it outsells even Prozac, the synthetic pill Americans began gobbling up in the late 1980s.

DR. DUKE'S NOTES

In some parts of the country, St. John's wort is better known by its common name, klamath weed. In California, where cattle have become photosensitive after grazing on large amounts of klamath, a movement has sprung up to eradicate the wild weed. There is even a monument, erected by the U.S. Department of Agriculture, to indicate success in biological control of the klamath weed in California. And, in 1998, California was having trouble supplying the demand for St. John's wort.

We're slow to catch on in America. Most of the studies showing hypericum's value as an antidepressant have been done abroad. In 1996, the *British Medical Journal* published an overview of 23 clinical studies, involving more than 1,700 patients. It concluded that hypericum has antidepressant properties, particularly in mild to moderate cases. And it said the herb was more effective than a placebo and just as potent as prescription antidepressants, without their side effects.

I'm almost positive I'm improving my emotional health by keeping St. John's wort on hand and using it when I feel the need.

Oddly, this herb has gained so much attention overseas, Ameri-

 HERB LORE AND MORE

Native Americans also turned to the healing qualities of St. John's wort, which early colonists brought to the New World. Interestingly, their uses are not the ones considered most effective today.

The Menominees compounded it with blackcap raspberry root and used it for kidney troubles. A compound containing the root was used to treat tuberculosis.

The Meskwakis applied a powder of the boiled root of St. John's wort to draw poison from the bite of the water moccasin. The Cherokees, too, chewed on the root, swallowing a portion and applying the rest as a poultice for snakebites.

The Cherokees took infusions of hypericum for fever and sniffed the crushed plant as a remedy for nosebleeds. Infusions also were used for bloody flux and bowel complaints. A compound decoction was taken to promote menstruation.

The Seminoles used infusion of roots for rat sickness and blocked urination and bowels. The Choctaw relied on a decoction of root for colic and as a wash for sore eyes.

The Miwok Indians depended on a decoction of the plant as a wash for running sores. It was thought to be a dermatological aid, perhaps because of its anti-inflammatory and antiviral properties, and it was used to break fevers and counteract venereal disease.

cans often are surprised when I tell them hypericum grows on its own in each of the 50 states. Early colonists likely brought it with them, either intentionally or by accident. Perhaps the tiny seeds hitched a ride on some food or other supply the settlers carried to the New World.

Thanks to our ancestors, you might have your own supply of this wonderful herb just down the road a bit or on your own soil, as I do. Although I never purposely cultivated St. John's wort until I established my Green Farmacy Garden in 1998, I suppose you could say it grew on me. The weed has a mind of its own in my garden, popping up wherever it likes, to heights of one to two feet, or three feet in an organic garden.

A Bountiful Garden and a Beautiful Bouquet

My wild-but-welcome St. John's wort includes *Hypericum perforatum* and *Hypericum punctatum*, 2 of about 400 species of the plant. My two happen to be among seven I studied in my years with the U.S. Department of Agriculture. All proved rich in at least one major active ingredient, hypericin, the focus of many studies.

Each year, around the third week of June, my plants bloom on schedule and continue to flower sporadically through first frost. (They may lapse into quiescence during droughts, only to liven up after the rains return.) It's as if they know I expect them. Their yellow petals are speckled with orange and reddish dots that ooze a purplish oil when pinched. Some herbalists liken the dots—where the active ingredients reside—to the pores of St. John's skin. When the flowers are steeped in oil, the "blood" in the pores moves into the oil. My *Hypericum punctatum* seems to have more of the purplish compounds. Just crushing it stains my fingers.

Sometimes, on summer strolls around my home, I gather the plants' flowering tops—so rich in phytochemicals. I could use them to make my own extract but generally prefer to take standardized capsules. That way, I know I'm getting the same amount of active ingredients with every dose—something I can't be sure of with the plants. Just like humans, each one of them is chemically unique.

St. John's wort also makes a beautiful bouquet. You probably can find the plants in summer at your local greenhouse. Although these commercially grown plants won't be as medicinally active, all St. John's wort seems to contain an aromatic called cineole. In studies, large quantities of cineole enabled rats to zip through a maze more rapidly, whether the compound was inhaled, applied to their skins, or force-fed to them.

Maybe a mere whiff of these mildly scented blooms can help us get happy. Why not place a pretty bouquet on a dining table or nightstand?

How St. John's Wort Can Help

St. John's wort contains dozens of active ingredients, such as hypericin, pseudohypericin, protohypericin, and hyperforin. Throughout history, myriad external and internal uses have been reported. Here are the ones I believe are the most scientifically sound:

Burns, cuts, and other wounds. Modern science backs up some of the folklore surrounding hypericum, including its ability to promote healing on our skin, not just underneath it.

Commission E has approved the topical use of St. John's wort oil for primary and secondary blunt and sharp injuries and for burns, skin damage caused by heat, caustics, electricity, or radiation. Hypericum is both an anti-inflammatory and antibiotic, which may help prevent infection. One study in Germany showed hypericum ointment speeded healing and lessened the severity of scarring.

Weed says the oil also reduces skin damage from radiation treatments. Women who applied the oil before and after treatments report their skin stayed healthy and flexible, even after dozens of exposures. Some suggest it may quicken healing from sunburn.

Depression. According to the World Health Organization, depression affects 3 to 5 percent of people. It's characterized by flagging mood, lack of interest in normally pleasurable activities, disturbed

A CASE IN POINT

Kimberly's Story

Can St. John's wort boost mood when combined with synthetic antidepressants?

The major pharmaceutical makers may not want to know. But plenty of folks who suffer from depression tell me they do—and some forward-thinking physicians are helping their patients find combinations that work.

Kimberly B., a fortysomething career woman in Virginia, who asked that her real name not be used, has fought mild but chronic depression since she was a teenager. "I thought I was lazy, until I learned in my late twenties what depression was," she says.

Kimberly says talk therapy helped her to "see differently," to view life's glass as half-full and not half-empty. She learned that depression could be hereditary. "A couple of my cousins have bipolar disorder," she says. "I think a couple of relatives struggled with alcoholism. They drank to deal with their depression."

Kimberly asked her doctor about synthetic antidepressants. "I wanted to know if I could feel better, the way normal people feel," she says. She tried commonly prescribed dosages of Prozac, then Zoloft, and then Paxil. But the side effects—nervousness, agitation, and irritability—wouldn't pass. Finally, with her doctor's help Kimberly settled on a "baby dose" of Luvox, a selective serotonin reuptake inhibitor (SSRI) used to treat obsessive-compulsive disorder and depression. Still, she says, the benefits seemed small.

Then, in 1997, Kimberly read the news reports about St. John's wort, and with her doctor's okay, began taking 300 milligrams containing 0.3 percent hypericin three times a day, in addition to the Luvox. (*Note:* I do not recommend combining hypericum with synthetic antidepressants without your doctor's approval.)

Kimberly says she noticed the effect almost right away. "In fact, by about the third day of using both, I felt overstimulated, so I cut back on the Luvox to every other day. Sometimes, I skip a dose or two of the St. John's wort. Otherwise, I haven't had any problems. I don't avoid any particular foods and, generally, I feel good."

eating and sleeping patterns, low self-esteem, indecisiveness, irritability, fatigue, and hopelessness.

In recent years, science has begun to shed light on depression—that its causes are environmental and biochemical, and that often it runs in families. We also have a new understanding of how depression occurs: through an imbalance in neurotransmitters, or feel-good chemicals such as serotonin, dopamine, and norepinephrine, which regulate mood.

This newfound knowledge has led to pharmaceuticals that target specific brain chemicals. One class of antidepressants called monoamine-oxidase inhibitors, or MAOIs, help raise the brain's supply of norepinephrine and dopamine. A newer class, selective serotonin reuptake inhibitors, or SSRIs, such as Prozac and Zoloft, ensure an abundance of serotonin.

DR. DUKE'S NOTES

While St. John's wort has been proven effective against unipolar depressions, evidence does not support its use in treating bipolar disorder, a condition in which sufferers "cycle" between depression and euphoria.

While studies show these Food and Drug Administration (FDA) approved drugs are effective for many, there is a price to pay—not only in dollars at the pharmacy but in side effects including dizziness, fatigue, dry mouth, constipation, and sexual dysfunction. Further, people taking the MAOIs must avoid certain foods and medications that interact with the drugs.

In the United States, Prozac is the best-selling antidepressant. But in Germany, about 200,000 prescriptions a month are filled for just one brand of St. John's wort, compared to about 30,000 a month for Prozac, says Varro E. Tyler, Ph.D., Sc.D., professor emeritus of pharmacognosy at Purdue University.

In German studies involving 3,250 people, 80 percent found partial or complete freedom from depressive symptoms, Dr. Tyler says in "The Honest Herbalist—The Secrets of Saint-John's-Wort," published in *Prevention* magazine.

In the United States, researchers are only beginning to study the herb's medicinal value. A three-year National Institute of Mental Health study at Duke University in North Carolina is comparing St. John's wort with Zoloft, or sertraline, the silver bullet in pharmaceu-

In Europe, hypericum has a long history as a treatment for depression, anxiety, and unrest. Research shows it boosts feel-good brain chemicals such as serotonin, dopamine, and norepinephrine.

For many years, it was believed hypericum acted primarily as a monoamine-oxidase inhibitor, or MAOI, enhancing dopamine and norepinephrine. The warning was given to avoid alcohol, smoked or pickled foods, and certain medications for allergies and colds, which might interact with hypericum, as with synthetic MAOIs.

Now, it appears the hypericum link was overplayed. My friend Jerry Cott, Ph.D., chief of the Pharmacologic Treatment Program at the National Institute of Mental Health, says the MAOI role is minor. It is more likely, as so often found in the plant world, that the compounds in St. John's wort work in synergy. They attack their opponent together, like a disciplined basketball team headed for the championship.

Consumers are likely to experience fewer side effects with the herbal remedy because of the shared actions of the compounds, says Varro E. Tyler, Ph.D., Sc.D., professor emeritus of pharmocognosy at Purdue University. Newer research on hypericum, for example, shows it also acts as a selective serotonin reuptake inhibitor (SSRI), increasing the mood-enhancing brain chemical serotonin.

I believe the empirically proven herbs are milder and safer because of this synergy. And their therapeutic effects may be more complete.

tical treatment of depression in this country. I am, like many, eager to see the results. These university trials satisfy something I have been urging for a decade: that new studies on pharmaceuticals compare them not only with placebo but also with a more promising herbal alternative. I'd like to see the FDA require that for every pharmaceutical so that we can see how the herbal remedy compares with the synthetic drug. But the FDA doesn't oversee herbal products, and there's little financial incentive for big drug manufacturers to test herbs, because they can't patent them. So my plea for mandatory comparisons with herbal alternatives as well as placebo remains unanswered. But the studies at Duke (no relation to myself) are at least one start in the right direction.

You'll most often see hypericin touted on St. John's wort product labels in the United States. But look for hyperforin, too. In Germany, newer studies are focusing on that chemical's action in the treatment of depression.

Herpes. St. John's wort may have antiviral benefits when applied topically to the oozing, painful blisters of genital herpes. The contagious viral infection affects about 45 million Americans, according to the National Institute of Allergy and Infectious Diseases (NIAID).

Herpes simplex II typically causes genital herpes, which is spread mainly through sexual contact with someone who has the virus. It lies dormant in the body between outbreaks. While oral and topical treatments can help reduce the number of outbreaks and their severity, there is no cure.

St. John's wort contains proven antivirals that can help speed healing when applied topically. It also can help heal cold sores and fever blisters caused by herpes simplex I, as well as the blisters of its cousins, chickenpox and shingles (varicella-zoster).

Shingles afflicts about 20 percent of adults who suffered a nasty, itchy bout of chickenpox in their earlier years. It is most common in people over 50. This virus, too, hides out in the body. When it erupts—often as the result of illness or stress—it causes pain and a blistering rash. The pain may linger for years after the visible sores have healed.

Hypericum contains analgesic properties that may help to quell the pain. If I had shingles, I would add a bit of capsaicin topically to my St. John's wort—but only after any open sores had healed.

Studies in the early 1990s showed hypericin is active against herpes simplex I and II. Herbalist Susun Weed also believes hypericum's antiviral powers pass through the skin and into the nerve endings, preventing and checking a variety of problems. She suggests hypericum internally (25 drops tincture) and externally, maybe every four hours, for shingles, cold sores, and genital herpes.

HIV/AIDS. The NIAID says as many as 900,000 Americans may be infected with human immunodeficiency virus, or HIV. It's the virus that causes AIDS, a major worldwide epidemic, first reported in the United States in 1981.

The virus kills or cripples the immune system's T-cells—the good guys—and leaves its victims unable to fight infection and certain cancers. They become susceptible to opportunistic infections, such as cytomegalovirus and herpes. In healthy people, the microbes that carry such infections don't usually cause illness. For people with HIV, they can be deadly.

HIV is passed along most commonly by sexual contact with an infected partner. The sharing of needles and syringes or contact with infected blood also can spread it. Mothers can transmit the virus to their babies during pregnancy or birth, NIAID says.

Some people have flu-like fever, headache, and fatigue a month or two after exposure. Severe symptoms may not occur for a decade or more. As the immune system weakens, signs such as swollen glands and weight loss begin to show. In advanced stages, HIV is categorized as AIDS. The virus can be detected by blood tests.

Standard treatments for HIV/AIDS include drugs such as AZT that interrupt an early stage of virus replication, slowing the virus in the body and delaying the onset of infections. Other drugs called protease inhibitors, such as saquinivir, interrupt the virus at later stages. Because HIV can become resistant to the drugs, often they are used in costly combinations, or drug "cocktails."

> **DR. DUKE'S NOTES**
>
> *Is it a placebo or is it hypericum? Clinical studies show a strong relationship between placebo pills and mood enhancement. In other words, people who think they are receiving medication may feel better, even if the pill is a dud. I'd rather "fool" myself with an herb than a costly pharmaceutical and the side effects that go with it.*

These cocktails can run as high as $18,000 a year. They require extreme diligence on the part of the patient, and they are not without side effects—nausea, diarrhea, and gastrointestinal disturbances among them. Patients must also be alert to signs of interaction with other drugs that can result in serious side effects, the NIAID acknowledges.

If I suffered from HIV/AIDS, I would also try the less expensive, safer herbal alternatives, including St. John's wort.

I first became curious about its role against HIV in the early

1980s. Gordon Cragg, Ph.D., at the Natural Products Branch of the National Cancer Institute (NCI), called and asked where we might be able to find hypericin. "In my garden," I told him. But it was September, past the plant's flowering season.

Daniel Meruelo, Ph.D., professor of pathology at New York University School of Medicine, wanted to examine the potential antiretroviral activities of hypericin in clinical trials. The AIDS connection was new to me, and exciting. The following spring I was able to supply them with hypericum.

 ## WHAT NEW RESEARCH TELLS US

Although more research must still be done, new studies are showing that St. John's wort may well be effective in dealing with a variety of health problems, including the following:

Obesity. Reports are that some antidepressants help curb appetite by increasing serotonin in the brain. That may be part of the reason the now infamous "fen-phen" drug combination pulled from the market in this country helped many dieters drop pounds. Studies now show hypericum acts on serotonin and likely a whole host of other brain chemicals. Some think it may prove helpful in the obesity battle. If Prozac can help curb obesity by increasing brain levels of serotonin, St. John's wort may have the same positive effect.

Smoking cessation. Research suggests cigarette smoking raises the brain's availability of the feel-good chemical dopamine—probably a major reason people find it so tough to quit. Some phytochemicals in hypericum also enhance dopamine in the brain. Maybe one day, smokers will give up their destructive weed with the help of this beneficial one, not inhaled but ingested.

Parkinson's disease. The dopamine connection may also prove beneficial in treating patients with Parkinson's disease. Researchers at the Brookhaven National Laboratory in Upton, New York, suggest it may be the now admittedly minor monoamine-oxidase inhibitor (MAOI) action of hypericum that plays a role. In test tube studies, they looked at a synthetic antidepressant, maclobemide, to show that when MAO is deficient, dopamine rises. Interestingly, the researchers report, smokers—perhaps by reducing MAO—have a lower risk for Parkinson's.

Dr. Meruelo was looking at hypericin in test tube studies, especially when combined with ultraviolet light. As with certain cancer treatments, researchers direct the tiny flashlight-like rays to hot spots where the virus is.

Dr. Cragg says hypericin itself did not appear to be the silver bullet in the NCI AIDS screen, but the work continues. Hypericum contains many ingredients that may help slow HIV. Dennis V.C. Awang, of the American Botanical Council Advisory board, has noted that pseudohypericin can reduce the spread of HIV, at least in the test

---

Arthritis and related swelling and pain. Oily hypericum preparations have anti-inflammatory activities that may be useful in treating arthritis, a rheumatic disease that causes pain, stiffness, and swelling of joints. Germany's Commission E (a panel of experts roughly equivalent to the U.S. Food and Drug Administration) heaps praise on St. John's wort, for external use, for myalgias (pain in one or more muscles). If I had arthritis, I'd certainly try the flowers, steeped in evening primrose, borage, and cod liver or olive oil as an external application. Hypericum oil also is popular in Germany as an external treatment for the pain and swelling of hemorrhoids.

Menopause and perimenopause. In an April 1999 media appearance, David Hnida, M.D., plugged St. John's wort for perimenopause, the six to eight years preceding menopause when a woman's ovaries stop producing eggs. Dr. Hnida says perimenopause is a hormonal transition phase that can leave women anxious and moody. They may have difficulty concentrating, sleeping, and remembering as well as they used to.

He recommends St. John's wort—whose phytochemicals work synergistically to affect mood—with the estrogens in clover or soy products, and the antioxidant vitamins A, C, and E. He also suggests perimenopausal women exercise, use alcohol in moderation, and quit smoking. Such advice carries right on through menopause. Research also shows hypericum can help with mood swings and depression that may result from hormonal changes. Many suggest it can help with premenstrual syndrome, or PMS, as well.

tube. At my urging, Jerry Cott, Ph.D., of NIMH may look at *Hypericum hypericoides*, yet another species. Hypericum also shows promise in fending off opportunistic infections, such as cytomegalovirus.

Hypericum might be doubly useful in treating AIDS because of its antiviral and antidepressant properties, says a 1995 article in the *Psychiatric Times*. The *Journal of the American Medical Association* reports that half of all people with a medical illness also are depressed. Adding St. John's wort to the HIV/AIDS weaponry might boost patient morale and the immune system, possibly slowing the virus.

Many more studies are needed before we know if hypericum can thwart HIV. It is not a cure. Unfortunately, "combination therapies" don't compare pharmaceuticals and St. John's wort for HIV, nor do any of the studies I have reviewed. But, if I had AIDS, I would certainly make the herb part of my daily routine along with antioxidants and immunostimulants to boost my immune system.

> ## DR. DUKE'S NOTES
>
> The oil from the crushed flowering tops of St. John's wort reportedly serves as a sunscreen, which I would not be afraid to use in my garden. That's ironic, given that St. John's wort raises the risk of photosensitivity or sunburn when ingested. In Europe, there have been reports of sheep suffering serious burns after grazing on large amounts of hypericum.

How to Take It and How Much

St. John's wort generally is available in capsules, tinctures, teas, and in bulk. For therapeutic use, I recommend standardized formulas. In general, follow the directions on the label. Here are some other guidelines, based on my experience:

Burns and cuts. Apply St. John's wort oil three or four times daily, as needed. Again, a cooled tea applied topically with cotton balls or a soft cloth also may be helpful.

Depression or seasonal affective disorder. Studies indicate a daily dose of 900 milligrams—containing 0.3 percent hypericin—may be useful. Also look on some labels for hyperforin, a phytochemical that is gaining attention in German studies.

Herpes. Brew a strong St. John's tea, let it cool, and apply it to the sores with a cotton ball. There may also be some value to using the hypericum internally, in capsules or tinctures. Finding an ointment containing hypericum is difficult in the United States, and it can be messy to make one.

HIV or AIDS. I would use a tincture made from the whole herb—about 10 to 30 drops in juice several times a day, along with other therapies my doctor recommended. I also would boost my immune system with daily doses of antioxidant supplements.

Useful Combinations

You may have seen over-the-counter hypericum supplements combined with kava kava, ginkgo biloba, and other herbal remedies. Do they work? There aren't any studies proving they do, but I don't think it's harmful to try them.

Exercise. Exercise and good nutrition go a long way toward balancing our moods. Andrew Weil, M.D., author of several books and the newsletter *Self Healing*, says aerobic exercise performed vigorously and often "is the best antidepressant." It increases production of endorphins, more of those mood-enhancing neurochemicals.

As a complement to hypericum and exercise, Dr. Weil recommends a few nutrients. Try 1,500 milligrams DL-phenylalanine (less if you have high blood pressure), 500 milligrams vitamin C, and 100 milligrams vitamin B_6 in the morning with fruit or juice about 45 minutes before breakfast. In the evening, add another 500 milligrams vitamin C and 100 milligrams B_6.

Light therapy. Sufferers of depression—and SAD, in particular—might also get relief by adding light therapy. Studies show a walk in daylight or regular sessions in front of a specially designed light box may increase levels of serotonin, norepinephrine, and other neurotransmitters that regulate mood. Watch out, though, for signs of photosensitivity.

Mood-enhancing teas. Making teas is a wonderful way to create your own designer herbs, one of my favorites for mood enhancement. For depression, Chris Hobbs, herbalist and author, suggests a tea of St. John's wort, damiana, lavender, rosemary, and wild oats. If I had HIV/AIDS, I'd try my All-Saints-Tea, combining any species of hypericum you can find and self-heal (*Prunella vulgaris*), sweetened with licorice.

Caution: Contraindications, Interactions, and Side Effects

St. John's wort is thoroughly safe for most users, but even so, certain people would do well to avoid combining it with some substances and to take precautions against possible side effects.

Sunworshippers. When supplementing with hypericum, wear sunscreen, and avoid overexposure to sun or ultraviolet light. Studies show St. John's wort can cause photosensitivity or sunburn, especially in the fair-skinned.

Pregnancy. Others will caution you not to use hypericum if you are pregnant. I have heard hints, though rare, of risks. I do not feel there is cause for serious concern, but do practice good judgment. I repeat here, as I will in almost all cases: If a pregnant woman needs an antidepressant, she and her physicians should weigh the risks of the herbal alternative, hypericum, versus the pharmaceutical one. More often than not, I'd probably vote for the herbal alternative. The same goes for lactating women and for children, even under two. If they need a drug, which is likely to do the most good with the fewest side effects, the herbal or the pharmaceutical?

Certain foods and alcohol. While the MAOI action of hypericum has been downgraded, I still would be cautious about using alcohol and pickled, smoked, or aged foods. Similarly, be careful about combining the herb with certain cold and hay-fever remedies (always read labels), amphetamines, tryptophan, or tyrosine. Another reason to avoid alcohol is that hypericum contains analgesics; studies show the two may interact.

Prescription drug alert. If you are taking an SSRI, such as Prozac or Zoloft, or any synthetic antidepressant, talk to your doctor about cutting back on the medication while beginning a regimen of St. John's wort. Some studies suggest too much serotonin can result in a condition called serotonin syndrome. Registered nurse Camilla Crachiolo reports that symptoms include confusion, fever, chills, sweating, and difficulty with speech. "It occurs most commonly when combining two antidepressants, but can occur with just one serotonin-increasing drug," she says.

A co-worker says she added hypericum supplements to the SSRI she takes for depression, under a doctor's care. She did, indeed, suffer side effects from the combination, but not what she expected. Rather than making her too "high," my colleague says the combination "mellowed" her out—almost too much.

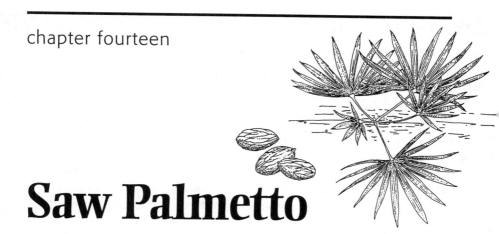

chapter fourteen

Saw Palmetto

LATIN NAME: *Serenoa repens*
FAMILY NAME: Arecaceae (palm family)

MAN'S BEST FRIEND is his dog, the old saw says. I'd like to add a Duke corollary: An old man's best friend may be his saw palmetto.

How could aging shift my allegiance from pooch to palm? Well, I figure a guy owes one helluva debt of gratitude to anything that, all by itself, averts prostate problems, may keep his hair from falling out, possibly bucks up his and his wife's libido and, on top of all of that, purportedly encourages breast growth.

Did the saw palmetto legend bring Ponce de León to Florida in search of the Fountain of Youth? I wonder. Maybe this small palm was actually the grail he held so holy.

What Saw Palmetto Is and What It Can Do

With fanlike, fingery fronds and small berry-shaped fruit, saw palmetto (*Serenoa repens*) grows naturally only in the Florida Everglades and certain other parts of the southeastern United States, maybe as far west as coastal Alabama and Mississippi and perhaps as far north as South Carolina.

Modern-day profiteers are trying to rewrite history by saying that

(continued on page 220)

The prostate gland, which only men have, secretes much of the fluid in semen. About the size of a walnut, it's located right above the rectum and encircles the urethra like a doughnut. As men age, the gland starts to grow, giving rise, sooner or later, to the condition called benign prostatic hyperplasia or benign prostatic hypertrophy (BPH). It's termed "benign" because the enlargement is not necessarily cancer-related nor necessarily associated with tumor growth. But it sure is problematic.

As the prostate enlarges, it chokes off the urethra and restricts the flow of urine. The larger the gland grows, the harder it becomes to urinate. Voiding becomes difficult, if not painful, and it's never completely successful. A man with full-blown BPH can't empty his bladder thoroughly, which explains one of BPH's telltale symptoms: frequent late-night trips to the bathroom. At its worst, BPH causes serious bladder and kidney problems, enough so to justify surgery.

An increased presence of the male hormone dihydrotestosterone (DHT), experts in urology and endocrinology generally concur, prompts the glandular growth by stimulating prostate cells to reproduce. DHT forms when the main male hormone, testosterone, interacts with an enzyme called 5-alpha-reductase.

Pharmaceutical companies spent millions and millions of dollars trying to come up with something that deterred 5-alpha-reductase and thus prevented the creation of DHT. (Don't applaud them for the expenditure; they've already recouped it.) Eventually, they concocted something called finasteride (sold under the brand name Proscar) that inhibits the body's release of 5-alpha-reductase. Without the enzyme, DHT levels drop, which allows the gland to shrink and improves BPH symptoms.

Holed up in laboratories holding up test tubes to Bunsen burners, scientists wasted a lot of time. Instead, they should've flown down to Florida, where they would have found a palm whose berries already contain such substances.

I don't like to chemically dissect a medicinal plant. You can identify hundreds of substances yet never be sure that any given one or ones may be responsible. In many cases, they may work best only when they work together. Some scientists have identified beta sitosterol, campesterol, stigmasterol, and other plant sterols as the key components. Others have cited free fatty acids and long-chain alcohols. Some Floridian scientists claim they've discovered as-yet unnamed sterols unique to saw palmetto, while others still have pointed fingers at one-of-a-kind acylglycerides with biological activity.

I don't doubt any of them. I think they're all correct. But they've all made *one similar mistake: They've sought to isolate one key component, and they've failed to realize that saw palmetto, like so many other herbal medicinals, is more than the sum of its chemical parts. Arguing over a specific compound in saw palmetto is an irrelevant diversion. The overriding issue is how saw palmetto, as an extracted whole, is better than anything the pharmaceutical industry has come up with.*

When the palm's active ingredients appear together in a standardized extract, they not only work as well as finasteride, they do finasteride one or two better. Besides inhibiting the 5-alpha-reductase enzyme, they block estrogens and already-created DHT from latching on to and affecting prostate cells. Other phytochemicals counter the tissue inflammation, which often occurs in BPH.

The natural medicine not only works on more levels than the synthetic, it works much quicker and works for a greater number of people. Proscar helps less than half of the men with BPH who take it, and they've got to wait at least six months before seeing some sign that it'll work at all.

Is All OK with the PSA?

Once saw palmetto emerged as the obvious, if uncrowned, treatment of choice for BPH, some critics counterattacked by charging that it interferes with a lab analysis, called the prostate-specific antigen (PSA) test, to detect a man's risk of prostate cancer. A higher measurement of this substance may indicate a higher risk of prostate cancer.

The evidence conflicts, so I can't give you a definitive answer. Some research asserts that taking saw palmetto has no effect whatsoever on PSA levels. Other research concludes that any inhibitor of 5-alpha-reductase, whether saw palmetto or finasteride or something else, theoretically should reduce PSA readings. If saw palmetto is guilty in this regard, finasteride is, too. Yet you never hear finasteride criticized for throwing off PSA readings. I wonder why?

And if this does indeed pose a problem, should men avoid eating vegetables entirely? To one degree or another, all plants contain PSA-reducing sterols. For instance, most beans contain genistein, an alpha-reductase inhibitor. Others include black-eyed peas, kudzu, lentils, soybeans, and split peas. Where is the advisory against eating these foods?

Again, no conclusive answer exists, but I'm not worrying about it. As long as you get a baseline PSA reading before you start to manipulate with herbs or pharmaceuticals, I think you'll be fine.

saw palmetto has always been a folk remedy for prostate problems. That's B.S. ("bum steer"), to put it bluntly. To Seminole Indians, the American saw palmetto was more of a food than a medicine. Only much later did people realize that its fruit encouraged urinary excretion and supported healthy genital function. Ironically, none of the traditional uses foreshadowed its current use.

In clinical trials, saw palmetto has beat the pants off its pharmaceutical rival, the synthetic drug finasteride (Proscar), for controlling the symptoms and possibly the cause of benign prostate enlargement. Benign prostatic hyperplasy or benign prostatic hypertrophy—BPH, as the condition is known—affects some 10 million American men every year. At least half of all 50-year-old men get it, and the older you grow from there, the more likely you'll be affected: At least 90 percent of all men 70 to 90 years old, by some estimates, must contend with BPH and its symptoms. About 30 percent of them eventually undergo surgery.

Head-to-Head

My mission in life is to force pharmaceutical companies to test their potions and notions directly against natural herbal alternatives. Head-to-head, one-on-one—let the best therapy win. I doubt that such even-handed contests will ever become standard operating procedure in my lifetime, but I'm winning battles here and there in this long war, and saw palmetto is one of the most glorious victories.

The triumphs are both professional and personal. According to the odds-makers, I should right now be one of some urologist's typical BPH patients. After all, as a 70-year-old, I carry about a 70 percent risk. But I do not have BPH.

Almost a decade ago, I decided to defy the long odds. In a wager made before a group of federal health officials, I bet my prostate gland that a preventive herbal approach was superior to finasteride, the first approved pharmaceutical treatment of choice for BPH. Since then, I've been beating ever-increasing odds.

At my most recent checkup, the doctor reported that my prostate was fine—neither seriously swollen nor inflamed, just slightly enlarged. "Whatever you're doing," he advised, "keep it up."

What I gambled on in the early 1990s is almost considered a safe bet today.

How Saw Palmetto Can Help

There is strong evidence supporting saw palmetto as a treatment for BPH and other conditions. The clinical trials establishing its therapeutic ability have been done in Europe, mostly Germany, where the palm is a primary urologic option. What Europe recognizes and what American medicine fails to accept is that even the stingiest of studies has found that saw palmetto is as effective as finasteride in relieving BPH. It is better tolerated and less likely to cause side effects.

The little American acknowledgment of the palm's efficacy has come belatedly and reluctantly. Witness a major 1998 analysis of saw palmetto's worth in mainstream medicine's biggest mouthpiece, *The Journal of the American Medical Association*. Investigators from the Minneapolis Veterans Affairs (VA) Medical Center reviewed 18 studies involving a total of 2,929 men with BPH. Even though the studies under scrutiny were positive, the VA scientists felt compelled to preface their findings with the qualifier that current saw palmetto research "is limited in terms of the short duration of studies and variability in study design, use of phytotherapeutic preparations, and reports of outcomes." But they couldn't avoid the inevitable conclusion for too long.

"However," they continued, "the evidence suggests that *S. repens* improves urologic symptoms and flow measures." In other words, it allows men with BPH to be better and pee better. The bottom-line determination of this comprehensive analysis? "Compared with finasteride, *S. repens* produces similar improvement in urinary tract symptoms and urinary flow and was associated with fewer adverse treatment events."

If I may translate: The herbal medicine is better than the drug, because it works just as well yet threatens users with less risk of side effects.

Because of how they work, both saw palmetto and finasteride do

A CASE IN POINT

What the Doctor Did

While writing this book, I sent some feelers out for good stories about saw palmetto. Christopher Hobbs, a third-generation medical herbalist and the author of a dozen or so very good books, including *Herbal Remedies for Dummies* and *Peterson's Field Guide of the Western U.S. Medicinals*, gave me a dandy.

Chris told me that his father, a long-time university professor and botanist, took the typical prescription route (finasteride) several years ago after recognizing certain prostate-related symptoms, specifically pain upon urination and the need to get out of bed some five to seven times a night to go to the bathroom. About a month after starting finasteride therapy, father called son to talk about side effects and therapeutic options.

"When I asked if he had changed his diet or medications at all," Chris said, "he told me about the new drug. I reviewed the side effects of Proscar, and they matched up perfectly."

Chris, a licensed acupuncturist in California, told his father to stop taking the medication. Instead, he said, take some saw palmetto extract. Chris sent his dad some supplements, and his dad took them faithfully.

After two months, the nighttime problems were no better, but at least all of the drug's side effects had vanished. Chris then decided his dad should double the dosage. Father followed son's orders. Three months later, Chris's dad called to say that the overnight urinary urges and inconveniences were gone. For the first time in untold months, he was able to sleep straight through the night.

This, in itself, is an excellent end to the story, but we're not quite done. There's a punch line.

You see, around the same time that the saw palmetto kicked into action,

carry a potential for adverse effects, specifically lowered libido, an inability to get an erection, a reduction in the amount of ejaculate, breast tenderness, and even breast growth (yes, in men as well as women). But there's a big difference between the *potential* for such adverse effects and their actual occurrence. Consequences of taking saw palmetto, the Minneapolis researchers noted, were "mild and in-

Chris's father went back to the doctor on an unrelated matter. "How are your prostate symptoms?" the physician asked, making conversation more than anything else during the course of the office visit. When the patient reported that all is now well, the doctor replied, "Great! Then the drug must have worked for you."

No, Chris's dad corrected, explaining that he had stopped taking the prescription drug nearly five months previously in favor of saw palmetto supplements.

"Oh," the doctor exclaimed. "I'm taking that, too."

An amusing anecdote? Sure. Ironic? You bet. A damned shame? Absolutely. Here is a doctor who prescribed a medication to his patient without informing him of an herbal alternative—an alternative that the doctor himself decided is the preferred option.

You and I are supposed to thrive in a society in which doctors are indoctrinated to give us certain authorized medications. They're not the safest medicines, and they're certainly not always the best. But they're almost always the most expensive. What do physicians know that they're not telling us about?

It's true that many doctors are reluctant to prescribe unapproved medicines for fear of litigation. The Food and Drug Administration (FDA) certainly doesn't help. Around the time that the agency approved finasteride, it also issued a warning and a reminder that saw palmetto was an unapproved therapeutic substance. Coincidence or biased conflict of interest?

Maybe we can't blame our nation's rank-and-file doctors for not telling their patients about the obvious superior treatment. But the FDA surely can't shrink from its role in steering American men in the wrong direction.

frequent." Among the study participants who took finasteride, 4.9 percent experienced erection difficulties; only 1.1 percent of the saw palmetto users suffered erectile problems.

A lot of other research is far more laudatory. Some studies, for instance, conclude that the average 320-milligrams per day dosage of the berry extract is three times stronger than the standard 5-milligrams per day dosage of finasteride. Other research found no significant statistical difference in how well either improved BPH symptoms. Finasteride resulted in a somewhat higher urinary flow compared with saw palmetto, but it also worsened sexual function.

This isn't the extent of the comparisons that can be made between saw palmetto and finasteride. Allow me to add two more:

➤ The phytochemical extract works faster and for more people. In sharp contrast to the man-made medicine, saw palmetto gets down to business in short order and works for a majority of the men who take it. In a strictly conducted German study, 88 percent of the men taking it and 88 percent of their physicians concluded that the berry extract was effective after just 90 days. Many of them noticed a considerable improvement in urinary symptoms after just a month and a half.

➤ On the other hand, you have to take Proscar for at least six months before noticing a significant benefit. What's more, you have less than a 50 percent chance that it'll work at all.

It's cheaper. Why shell out more money for something that doesn't work as well as its competition and poses more of a potential for harm? Prices vary from city to city around the country, but a year's worth of saw palmetto, according to one estimate, runs up to about $180. A year's worth of finasteride, in contrast, sets you back some $600—more than three times as much money. Hytrin, another pharmaceutical for BPH that works by a different mechanism, costs about $460 a year.

Surgery to relieve the urinary obstruction of an enlarged prostate can run you many thousands of dollars. Though the number of these operations has declined as finasteride sales have skyrocketed, the procedure is still one of the most common reasons men over the age of 65 go under the knife.

The operation, called transurethral resection of the prostate (TURP), often doesn't work. A study of 400,000 men who had a TURP found that they are more likely to require additional prostate surgery in five years than are men who stayed clear of the operating room. They're also more likely to die than men who had the more serious prostatectomy surgery. And some 6 percent of TURP patients end up impotent.

All in all, BPH management is a $3-billion-a-year business. How much of that, do you suppose, represents purchases of saw palmetto supplements? Are these guys getting their money's worth, or are they getting ripped off?

Hair regrowth. Having apparently won my initial wager, I'm taking my gambler's luck from my prostate to my pate. I'll bet my hair that saw palmetto curbs the hair loss of male pattern baldness and promotes regrowth at least as well as mainstream medicine's favored pharmaceutical.

You see, a funny thing happened on the way to testing finasteride's impact on benign prostate enlargement: A lot of study participants noticed the return of lost hair—or at least a significant slowdown or halt in the rate of balding. Further research using much smaller amounts of finasteride (1 milligram a day, as opposed to 5 milligrams) confirmed the reports. Ultimately, pharmaceutical marketing put a different suit on an old chemical and presented a hot new drug, Propecia, backed with its own multimillion-dollar ad campaign.

The science behind the treatment apparently makes sense. Male pattern baldness, most specialists agree, stems from the activity of certain male hormones in the scalp, specifically the presence of that old bugaboo dihydrotestosterone. It's formed when the 5-alpha-reductase enzyme interacts with testosterone. If this mechanism is indeed responsible for baldness, then whatever inhibits the enzyme down below should work up top, too.

That brings us back to saw palmetto. We know that it inhibits 5-alpha-reductase at least as well as (perhaps better) and unquestionably more safely than finasteride, no matter what drug dosage you use (and no matter what pharmaceutical brand name you might give it).

I've collected a handful of anecdotal accounts that the berry extract does trigger renewed hair growth on your head. While in Los Angeles to promote my book, *The Green Pharmacy*, for instance, I met a radio announcer who told me that taking it had helped to restore hair he lost from a prescription hormone treatment. A few middle-aged gardeners at my herbal vineyard can also doff their caps and point to very fine hair regrowth that's characteristic of finasteride use but apparently is prompted by saw palmetto. They weren't on the drug. They were on saw palmetto.

Other uses. Over the ages, folk medicine practitioners have used saw palmetto for a diverse range of health complaints. None of these

 ## HERB LORE AND MORE

Breast enlargement is just one of saw palmetto's traditional hormone-related applications. According to the 1898 edition of *King's American Dispensatory*, it's been used for ovarian enlargement associated with tenderness and pain, low libido, sterility, impotence, and dysmenorrhea, or menstrual cramps. Its berries are also said to ease uterine irritability, stimulate urination, and spark growth in "wasted organs," such as the ovaries and testes.

Today, we have a multimillion-dollar plastic surgery industry, but a century ago, all we had was saw palmetto. The palm was our best-known folk treatment to enlarge a woman's breasts. Naturopathic doctors still suggest it for this purpose.

Does it work? I'm not so certain that saw palmetto is the best plant for more mammary mass. Then again, who am I to argue with satisfied customers? A woman from North Carolina called me out of the blue one day to tell me that after reading my book, *The Green Pharmacy*, she started to take both saw palmetto and fenugreek to enlarge her breasts. Though she stopped taking the latter herb because she read that it worked hormonally (actually, both work via a hormonal mechanism), she continued to take saw palmetto. And her top measurement did indeed increase.

She is one of three women who have offered unsolicited testimonials to the bust-blooming power of the palm since *The Green Pharmacy* was published. I've also had three unsolicited offers from supplement manufacturers seeking endorsements for newly created mammary enhancers. And one account that

other treatments has been verified by science, although some make sense based on the fruit's phytochemical content.

The berries are said to support the entire male reproductive system, stimulating genital blood flow and improving the thyroid gland's regulation of sexual development. For women, the fruit supposedly alleviates ovarian and uterine irritations and cystitis. It purportedly triggers breast growth and lactation, too.

Regardless of gender, saw palmetto has been used for kidney problems, diarrhea, bronchitis, digestive difficulties, fluid retention, nasal congestion, and lack of appetite. Its berries also supposedly ease

I've read cites the patient experiences of three different practitioners who attest to the palm's breast-building ability.

For a so-called "mastogenic" herb, better scientific justification and more anecdotal evidence falls on the side of fenugreek, although it has a better reputation for encouraging milk secretion than for prompting the need for a larger bra. But in tests on lab animals, one of the plant's active ingredients, diosgenin, indeed stimulated breast growth.

Other lactation-inducing herbs from folklore include alfalfa, anise, basil, caraway, celery root and seed, chickpea, dill, fennel, Iceland moss, kudzu, lettuce, lemon balm, marjoram, nutsedge, okra, pea, purslane, sesame, sponge gourd, and verbena. I'm sure many of them will show up in new "bus-teas" as entrepreneurs capitalize on ostensible alternatives to silicone.

The only one I'd put money down on is fenugreek; of the others, all I can say is that some of them might help enhance fenugreek's flavor. I've read elsewhere that subcutaneous injections of reserpine, a compound in Indian snakeroot that lowers blood pressure, increases mammary gland secretions in rabbits.

If I had discovered the secret to natural breast enlargement and a stronger libido, I'd be hobnobbing in Hollywood, not meandering about in a suburban Maryland garden. I'm still meandering in that Maryland garden—and loving every minute—so take these possibilities for what they're worth.

anxiety. In recent years, bodybuilders and weightlifters have been taking saw palmetto supplements, reasoning that the plant's ability to preserve testosterone will allow them to increase muscle mass.

How to Take It and How Much

It goes without saying that you want to take a standardized extract. That's what I do. Depending on the concentration in the brand you select, you'll need to take anywhere from 150 to 1,200 milligrams per day. A product that contains 90 percent fatty acids and sterols is a good strength. The higher the concentration of sterols, the lower the dosage.

Other forms of saw palmetto, in my opinion, are neither strong enough nor economically feasible. You might need to take between ½ and 2 grams thrice daily of the dried whole fruit, 0.6 to 1.5 milliliters of a liquid fruit extract, or 5 to 6 milliliters of a liquid whole-herb extract. Another option is to brew the dry powder into a tea. Be forewarned, though: As much as I treasure my own saw palmetto (a birthday present from daughter Cissie), the fruit tastes most unpleasant. It stinks, too. I trust the wisdom of the Seminole Indians implicitly, but I can't for the life of

---

DR. DUKE'S RECIPES

Prostnut Butter

If speed, taste, fuss, and muss are of no concern, you might want to whip up a batch of my "Amazonian Prostnut Butter" cracker and sandwich spread, full of foods that also have prostate-protecting properties.

To make my spread, load the blender with about 10 medium-sized Brazil nuts, 50 to 100 pumpkin seeds, ½ cup of bean sprouts (I prefer black beans to soybeans), and a few sun-dried tomatoes or a little tomato paste. For the saw palmetto, I blend in a small handful of whole seeds, but you'll find it easier just to sprinkle in the contents of a capsule or two. Don't make a big batch, only enough for a few days. You want fresh phytomedicine.

Eat a couple of tablespoons a day, or spread it on a piece of bread or some crackers. I like to chase it down with a glass of either tomato juice, pink grapefruit juice, or watermelon juice. Each gives you lycopene's antioxidant and antiprostatic protection.

me figure out how they ate this stuff. Their palates and yours may differ from mine.

Useful Combinations

As potent as saw palmetto appears to be, you can further maximize your prostate protection and further multiply your chance of deterring hair loss with the assistance of many other medicinal plants.

In parts of Europe, phytomedicine is the preferred first course of action against BPH. In Germany and Austria, physicians use therapeutic plant extracts to treat some 90 percent of all mild and moderate cases. That accounts for about 90 percent of all drugs prescribed for the condition.

In Germany alone, more than half of all urologists turn first to phytochemicals for mild to moderate forms of BPH. Of the $160 million spent yearly on prostate medicine, 80 percent goes to herbal alternatives, mostly saw palmetto, pumpkin seeds, nettle root, and rye pollen. Each of these natural alternatives, by the way, comes with the blessings of the Commission E (a German panel of experts roughly equivalent to the U.S. Food and Drug Administration). In Italy, plant extracts represent 49 percent of all pharmacological BPH treatments.

Prostate Problems

The American medico-pharmaceutical industry is depriving you of some darned good therapies for benign prostate enlargement. Here's what you're missing:

Brazil nuts. If the prostate benefits from an antioxidant sentry, then the Brazil nut is just the guard for the job. The average nut contains a whopping 70 micrograms of selenium and is rich in vitamin E and prostate-friendly sterols.

Gamma linolenic acid (GLA). While attending a conference in Scotland a few years ago, my assistant learned from a leading British urologist, Dr. A. Colin Buck, that this essential fatty acid employs the same mechanism as saw palmetto to deter the hormone responsible for prostate enlargement. The combination of GLA and saw palmetto, the urologist said, holds great potential to alleviate BPH.

You'll find GLA in evening primrose oil, black currant oil, and borage oil. I prefer evening primrose, as explained in chapter 6.

Licorice. True licorice also contains a substance that inhibits the formation of dihydrotestosterone, although the therapeutic influence may come with a cost. I've never noticed any ill effects, but some people, after taking large doses for a long time, get headaches, retain fluid, and become lethargic, among other problems. If you're not prone to hypertension or low potassium, I doubt that reasonable doses would spell trouble for you. Nevertheless, keep your eyes open.

*Pumpkin (*Cucurbita pepo*).* Now here's a long-standing treatment for age-related prostate enlargement. Too bad that *another* American plant became a traditional remedy not on these shores but in Europe, particularly Turkey, Bulgaria, and the Ukraine.

Pumpkin seeds apparently act as a diuretic, which partly explains the better urinary flow men seem to notice after ingesting them. Pumpkin phytochemicals also appear to protect prostate cells from the gland-growing hormone dihydrotestosterone. In one study, BPH patients took 90 milligrams of isolated pumpkin sterols before undergoing surgery to remove their prostates. Tissue analyses later confirmed that the pumpkin users' glands contained less dihydrotestosterone.

Other researchers speculate that two antioxidant nutrients, alpha-tocopherol (vitamin E) and the mineral selenium, protect the gland. Naturopaths, meanwhile, attribute the therapeutic activity more to the abundant presence of three amino acids—alanine, glycine, and glutamic acid. Eating a handful of pumpkin seeds probably provides more than the 10-gram (one-third ounce) dosage that Germany's Commission E recommends. That handful, by the way, gives you more than the 200 milligrams of each amino acid that naturopaths usually suggest.

Pygeum. Some call it the Malagasy Medicinal Tree, while others know it as the African cherry, among many other names. Whatever you call it, pygeum is a relatively new kid on the prostate block, but it's made an impressive debut. Of pygeum users in a German study of almost 250 men, 66 percent enjoyed an improvement in BPH symptoms, compared to those who took a placebo. Other research suggests that the tree's bark is best for quelling glandular inflammation and improving sexual performance among men with prostate disease.

Stinging nettle (Urtica dioica). This folk medical anti-arthritic and diuretic also is relatively new to prostate protection. In a small clinical study of 67 men over the age of 60 with prostate cancer, taking a nettle extract relieved nighttime urinary problems. Other research shows that a root extract protects prostate cells from certain hormonal substances aside from the one that causes glandular growth. It's also an anti-inflammatory. Germany's Commission E okayed nettle not for prostate cancer or prostatitis per se but for urinary problems stemming from the diseases.

Tomato. If, as we suspect, antioxidant activity helps protect the prostate, then lycopene from tomatoes must surely be part of the team. This free-radical fighter, found predominantly in tomatoes (cooked are better than raw), also possesses proven prostate-protecting qualities. A study I heard about on CNN a few years ago found that men who ate tomatoes four to seven times a week had 20 percent fewer cases of prostate cancer. Those who dined on "love apple" 8 to 20 times a week had a 45 percent smaller incidence of the disease.

Hair-Loss Helpers

My hairline has formed itself into a prominent widow's peak over the years, but it hasn't crawled back to my crown. Who knows what's responsible for causing (or preventing) that. What I do know is that no one has a cure for baldness right now. Still, I'd put my money down on a saw palmetto herbal hair tonic before any of Propecia's prescription promises—or any other herbal tonic, for that matter. For male pattern baldness, saw palmetto is the only one I'd bet on. Given the similar methods of action, licorice and stinging nettle might help, too, but I just don't know. Other "farmaceutical follicle fertilizers" are certainly worth a try, but I suspect they are not much better (or worse) than any other over-the-counter hair nostrum you might find.

Aloe. You might start with the heralded burn plant. It might take the aloe out of alopecia. With phytochemicals that heal and replenish skin tissue, aloe vera has proved useful against acne, dandruff, seborrhea, and other dermatological problems.

Danshen. Here's another traditional hair protectant, found in many shampoos and rinses. Besides stemming hair loss, it purportedly prevents graying.

Other herbs. Innumerable other herbs, nutrients, and natural nostrums supposedly save and maintain your mane, including forsythia, fo-ti, ginger, horse chestnut, horsetail, mume, rosemary, safflower, and sesame. Don't get your hopes up, though. I'm skeptical about whether any medicine, natural or synthetic, can treat all causes of hair loss. The best we seem able to do is redress male pattern baldness. And when it comes to that, saw palmetto, in my "mental pharmacopoeia," is the drug of choice.

Caution: Contraindications, Interactions, and Side Effects

Men concerned about BPH usually don't have to worry until they've reached the age of 40. After that, saw palmetto becomes a definite preventive option, but don't start to take supplements until you've talked to a doctor or urologist and have had a baseline measurement of your PSA (prostate-specific antigen) levels.

Given that one of the several ways in which saw palmetto works is the same as finasteride's method of action, the standardized supplement should probably carry the same precautions and contraindications as the drug. Note that I said "probably." All of the clinical trials concluded that the berry extract was better tolerated by more people. Side effects cropped up only infrequently and, when they did occur, were mild.

Erection-related problems. According to calculations by the VA researchers, 1.1 percent of saw palmetto users noticed erection-related difficulties, compared with 4.9 percent of the men taking finasteride.

Nature, in its infinite, innate wisdom, abides by Hippocrates' first dictum. First, do no harm. However, I feel obligated to state that the side effects of finasteride—and thus saw palmetto—include a reduction in sex drive, an impaired ability to get an erection, and a drop in the amount of ejaculate. Not all studies have recorded all of these side effects. Some are even contradictory. Researchers have also noted an *enhancement* in sexual arousal. Sadly, despite the unusual number of clinical trials involving saw palmetto, we still don't know everything we should know about this herbal medicine.

Breast tenderness and enlargement. This is a condition called gynecomastia. Yes, I'm afraid, some men might notice a little fatty growth around their nipples. The risk supposedly increases the longer you take the supplement.

Pregnancy alert. I especially don't know what to make of one of finasteride's primary warnings: that pregnant women and women who are even thinking about conceiving shouldn't even touch a tablet. The reason is that female lab animals that were pregnant or became pregnant when taking finasteride gave birth to male babies with deformed genitalia. Does saw palmetto pose the same peril? Again, we simply don't know.

chapter fifteen

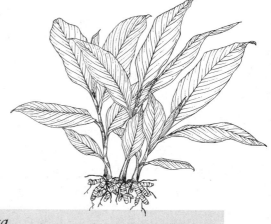

Turmeric

LATIN NAME: *Curcuma longa*
FAMILY NAME: Zingiberaceae

YOU MAY RECOGNIZE turmeric as the spice that's widely used in Indian cuisine. Native to India and tropical areas of Asia, it's what gives curry powder its vibrant yellow hue. It's also the ingredient that makes American-style mustard so yellow.

Turmeric is made from the root of *Curcuma longa*, a beautiful tropical plant with yellow or yellowish-white flowers, luscious fruits, and very large lilylike leaves.

Its exotic fragrance once made the flowers a favorite for making fragrances. And herbal healers have been using it for thousands of years to stop inflammation.

I'm hopeful that taking turmeric and its anti-inflammatory relatives, ginger and cardamom, will help protect me from the type of arthritis that ruined the last decade of my mom's life. The arthritis permanently locked her right arm into a dysfunctional curve, a painful and debilitating condition that eventually repeated itself on her left side.

In her last years, the arthritis robbed her of her independence. This certainly will not do for me, addicted as I am to my guitar playing.

What Turmeric Is and What It Can Do

The leaves of turmeric generally aren't used. Ordinarily, only the rhizomes, or roots, are used for medicinal purposes and for food flavoring. Turmeric is harvested at the end of the growing season and sun dried. Herbalists usually use dried roots, although sometimes they stew them instead. They call this "guisador" in Peru but "azafran" elsewhere in Latin America.

One secret of turmeric's medicinal power is the many antioxidants it contains. You'll recognize some of the more common ones, such as vitamins C and E, along with several carotenoids. It also contains lesser-known, but more effective antioxidants—specifically, curcumin and related compounds called curcuminoids.

Recently, substances called cyclooxygenase inhibitors have won praise as powerful miracle aspirins for blocking inflammation, especially inflammation caused by arthritis and, my own personal affliction, gout (gout is a type of arthritis). Turmeric, like its cousin ginger, contains some natural cyclooxygenase inhibitors. Some studies compare it to ibuprofen. Research suggests it works almost as well and with none of the side effects.

In fact, studies also suggest that turmeric can stop inflammation about half as well as a corticosteroid called cortisone. Corticosteroid medications are considered the "gold standard" for stopping inflammation. The problem with these drugs is that their potential side effects, such as fluid retention, high blood pressure, and bone damage, are nearly as impressive as their benefits. Given a choice, I'll go with the more natural (and flavorful) "gold standard" turmeric any day.

How Turmeric Can Help

I'm a big believer in the anti-inflammatory benefits of turmeric But it has many other uses as well. That's the great thing about this herb: When you take it for

It makes perfect sense to me that turmeric, with its rich supply of curcumin, works so well as an anti-inflammatory. Research has shown that this compound inhibits the body's production of certain prostaglandins, hormonelike substances of which some play a direct role in causing inflammation.

What's so exciting about turmeric is that it appears to target specific "inflammatory pathways" in the body.

In other words, it targets some prostaglandins, but not all of them. This is important because a targeted approach helps give the benefits with much fewer risks of side effects.

To understand how turmeric works, you have to understand a little bit about the inflammatory process. There are two basic types of prostaglandins: cyclooxygenase-1 (COX-1) and cyclooxygenase-2 (COX-2). The body needs COX-1 prostaglandins to function normally. Among other things, these substances help blood clot properly. COX-2 prostaglandins, on the other hand, are only produced in response to inflammation, such as that caused by arthritis.

Traditional medications such as aspirin block the body's production of both types of prostaglandins. While this certainly stops swelling, it also interferes with the normal levels of COX-1. This is why people taking aspirin may have trouble with bleeding—the blood isn't able to clot the way it should. This isn't a minor problem. Scientists estimate that about 20 percent of people who could benefit from these drugs can't take them because of the risk of gastrointestinal bleeding.

There was a great deal of excitement in the scientific world when researchers developed a medication that selectively blocked the COX-2 pathway. This made it possible to stop inflammation without affecting the blood's natural ability to clot. This is indeed an important medical breakthrough—but herbalists have been getting the same result all along by using turmeric and ginger, which may possibly target the same pathway.

In fact, a variety of herbs and plants do the same thing. On the same day I read the news about the new medication, I also discovered that weedy plantains, traditionally used for inflammation, contain two COX-2 inhibitors, ursolic acid and oleanolic acid. I'll bet that we'll soon hear that most anti-inflammatory herbs contain one or more of these specialized compounds.

one thing, you automatically afford yourself protection against many other problems, some of them quite serious.

Athlete's foot. I usually prevent this itchy fungal infection by the simple expedient of going barefoot. But should this stop working and I find myself with itchy feet, I apply a paste made from turmeric—or, in some cases, ginger, a close relative of turmeric that may be even more effective. Both ginger and turmeric pastes appear to destroy the guilty fungus. Garlic works too.

Speaking of annoying foot conditions, I also recommend turmeric for bunions, those painfully inflamed deformities that occur on the side of the foot or big toe. Its anti-inflammatory action helps reduce the swelling that makes bunions so painful.

Cancer. There is good evidence to suggest that turmeric helps prevent colon, breast, and lung cancers as well as melanomas (and you may recall from earlier chapters that I'm genetically targeted for colon cancer). In animal studies, for example, researchers have found that turmeric—or, more specifically, the curcumin it contains—may reduce the risk of colon cancer by 58 percent. One reason it's so powerful is that it interferes with at least four separate links in the cancer-causing chain.

For starters, curcumin appears to literally neutralize some cancer-causing substances. After that, it acts as an antimutagenic, meaning it stops very early changes in cells that can turn to cancer. At still later stages, curcumin appears to reduce the number and size of different types of tumors. Importantly, curcumin also possesses antimetastatic properties.

Digestive complaints. I'm convinced that the curcumin in turmeric exerts a number of beneficial effects in the gastrointestinal tract. Research suggests that it helps increase the mucous content in gastric juices, which can make it helpful for stomach disorders. Some herbalists say that turmeric should not be used by people with gallbladder disease, but I believe there is pretty solid evidence that it can increase bile flow and actually help disintegrate gallstones.

ALL IN THE FAMILY: CARDAMOM

A turmeric cousin, cardamom is an aromatic spice often used to flavor stews and curries. It traces its origins to southern India and Sri Lanka, and it's also cultivated in Southeast Asia and Guatemala.

What Cardamom Is and What It Can Do

Medicinally, cardamom has been used in Asia as an aphrodisiac. In Arab countries, coffee houses often mix some into coffee. I cannot verify its effectiveness in this particular regard, but cardamom does contain a compound called cineole, which stimulates the central nervous system—and I suppose this could give thoughts of romance a little boost. Cineole is often used by aromatherapists as a remedy for fainting. I like to spike my coffee or tea with a couple of seeds.

How Cardamom Can Help

Cineole is an antiseptic that can kill bad breath bacteria, which may explain in part its reputation as an aphrodisiac. Try chewing on a few seeds, then spitting them out.

Like spearmint, rosemary, eucalyptus, ginger, bee balm, peppermint, and other herbs with high cineole content, cardamom makes a great expectorant for people with laryngitis. Make a tea combining these ingredients, and add some pineapple juice.

Cardamom has also been found to be effective for eliminating, or at least limiting, gas. A few sprinkles on a piece of toast may do the trick as well as the cinnamon that my wife uses.

How to Take It and How Much

Cardamom is available as seeds, oil crushed from seed, and as a tincture, standardized to 1 to 2 grams as cineole. A recommended daily dosage of tincture is 1.5 grams standardized as cineole. If you take the proper dosage, you should be free of any health hazards or side effects.

In one study, mice with experimentally induced gallstones were fed modest amounts of turmeric. Within 5 weeks their gallstone volume had dropped by 45 percent, and after 10 weeks, by 80 percent.

Because curcumin increases the solubility of bile, it may help prevent gallstones from forming. If I had gallstones, I would definitely cook lots of curries—and go heavy on the turmeric. But some herbalists would disagree. Not me.

Heart disease. The antioxidants in herbs and foods are among the most powerful tools for protecting the heart. This is because they help prevent the oxygen in the body from damaging (oxidizing) molecules of cholesterol in the blood stream. This is important because cholesterol that's been oxidized may cause plaque and potential blockage, making it more likely to impede the flow of blood to the heart. Since curcumin is a potent antioxidant, I'm convinced that it can help prevent cholesterol from causing the narrowing of the arteries, called atherosclerosis, that's among the main causes of heart attacks.

Turmeric helps the heart in another way, as well. It appears to help prevent tiny cell-like structures in blood, called platelets, from clumping together and causing clots.

HIV. The evidence is still preliminary, but I think it is more than worthwhile for people who are HIV-positive to include as much turmeric in their diets as they can stand. Curcumin is believed to have antiviral properties, along with antilymphomic properties that could be useful to HIV patients.

Liver problems. I strongly recommend that people who have been exposed to environmental toxins, such as the pesticide DDT and the environmental pollutants 4-nonylphenol and 4-octylphenol, add a lot of extra turmeric to their diets. Turmeric steps up the production of three enzymes—aryl-hydrocarbon-hydroxylase, glutathione-S-transferase, and UDP-glucuronyl-transferase. These are chemical "knives" that break down potentially harmful substances in the liver. Turmeric offers similar protection for people who are taking medications such as methotrexate and other forms of chemotherapy, which are metabolized by, or shuttled through, the liver.

While I don't expect anyone to remember these long, tongue-twisting names, I do think it is fascinating that one little herb can strong-arm so many different chemicals. That's the ever-amazing power of the food farmacy.

Skin problems. Turmeric doesn't have to be taken internally to be effective. It also helps reduce inflammation, such as that caused by acne, when it's ground into a powder and applied as a poultice to the skin.

Wound healing. Whenever you have a cut, the body responds by flooding the area with immune cells and fluids. While this process helps clean the area and prevent infection, it can also cause painful swelling and inflammation, which slows the time it takes wounds to heal. By blocking this process, turmeric (and the curcumin it contains) can help wounds heal more quickly. In laboratory research at the Center for Combat Casualty and Life Sustainment Research in Bethesda, Maryland, scientists found that animals given curcumin healed much faster than those who weren't given the extra protection.

How to Take It and How Much

I'm all for enjoying turmeric in fabulous food. One of the most palatable approaches to treating arthritis, for example, is with curries—as long as you really load on the turmeric.

Supplements. I like turmeric a lot, but I don't want to eat it every day. For most people it's easiest to take the main active ingredient, curcumin, in supplements. I recommend taking 1,200 milligrams daily, divided into three doses. You can buy capsules that contain 400 to 450 milligrams.

(continued on page 244)

Dioscorides, the "surgeon general" to the Roman emperors Claudius and Nero, wrote that ginger "warms and softens the stomach." More than 2,000 years later, researchers continue to recommend ginger for stomach complaints, especially nausea.

What Ginger Is and What It Can Do

Ginger is an amazing plant. It grows up to 3 feet tall and has thick, knotty underground stems called rhizomes. These gnarled rhizomes, known as ginger root, contain a powerful class of compounds called gingerols. Gingerols appear to give digestive relief by inhibiting intestinal spasms. Ginger's zingibain, a type of enzyme that breaks down protein, may be responsible for its anti-inflammatory properties.

Herb Lore and More

Ginger gets its name from the Sanskrit word meaning "horn-shaped"—a name that won't come as a surprise to anyone who has ever seen the root. It was one of the most abundantly used spices in the Middle Ages; historians say that practically every sauce recipe included it.

Western herbalists use the dried and fresh forms of ginger interchangeably. According to traditional Chinese medicine, however, each form has different uses.

Fresh ginger, called *sheng-jiang*, is usually recommended for cold symptoms such as coughing, chills, and sneezing. Dried ginger, called *gan-jiang*, is used for a wider range of conditions, including digestive complaints, menstrual problems, immune disorders, and food poisoning. Apart from the great taste, this is one reason the Chinese use ginger to season seafood dishes. If the fish happens to be contaminated, the addition of ginger may help neutralize its harmful effects.

How Ginger Can Help

When I get a cold, I make lots of strong ginger tea, using a few tablespoons of fresh, shredded ginger root. It's a sensible thing to do, because ginger contains nearly a dozen antiviral compounds. Known as sesquiterpenes, these compounds are especially effective at fighting the family of viruses known as rhinoviruses—the organisms that cause colds.

But ginger has a wide variety of uses, and it's particularly effective for digestive complaints. Its chemical compounds soothe the digestive tract and aid digestion by increasing peristalsis, the wavelike muscle contractions that move food through the intestine. This in turn helps control diarrhea and intestinal cramps. Commission E (a German panel of experts roughly equivalent to the U.S. Food and Drug Administration) approves taking two grams (one teaspoon) of ginger in tea for indigestion.

Perhaps ginger has received the most attention, however, for its role in quelling motion sickness. In one study, 36 people were divided into groups. Those in one group were given 940 milligrams of dried ginger. Those in the second group were given dimenhydrinate, the active ingredient in over-the-counter motion-sickness remedies. People in both groups were then blind-folded and put in a spinning chair. Those given the ginger were able to withstand 5½ minutes in the chair before getting sick. Those taking the medication only lasted 3½ minutes. Ginger, in other words, was 57 percent more effective than medication in forestalling that awful queasy feeling we've all experienced from time to time.

This study was impressive, but other researchers have had mixed results. I think this is because there's considerable variability in the quality of commercial ginger preparations. Evidence also suggests that timing is critical. Ginger seems to be most effective when it's taken at least four hours before a trip.

In addition to its role in treating motion sickness, ginger might be useful for stopping the nausea associated with chemotherapy or the use of anesthesia during surgery.

How to Take It and How Much

There aren't any definitive studies showing how much ginger you need to get the best results. Specialists in herbal medicine usually suggest using 1 to 2 grams of powdered ginger—the equivalent of 10 grams (about 1 tablespoon) of fresh ginger, 2 teaspoons of ginger syrup, or 2 milliliters of ginger extract.

When you're buying ginger supplements, liquids, or powders, look for products that have a standardized dose of 20 percent (about 200 milligrams) gingerol. If you like the taste of ginger, however, it's easy to get all you need by using fresh root or powder. People in India, for example, eat an average of 8 to 10 grams of ginger a day.

Caution: Contraindications, Interactions, and Side Effects

Ginger is reportedly contraindicated for morning sickness and should not be taken by anyone with gallstones.

If you really like turmeric, you'll get similar effects by using the herb itself. However, you'll have to take a lot—up to 6 or 8 teaspoons a day. That's an amount most people will find a little difficult to get down.

Dried root. The recommend dose is 1.5 to 3 grams a day.

Oil. To get rid of the burning and itching of athlete's foot, I recommend using oil of turmeric. Dilute one part oil to two parts of water and apply it directly to the affected area, using a cotton ball or clean cloth.

Poultice. An excellent way to relieve the pain of bunions is to apply a teaspoon of fresh, grated turmeric to the bunion twice a day. The poultice acts directly on nerve endings at the site of trouble. It reduces the amount of substance P, a pain-transmitting chemical, that's produced by the nerves. Turmeric, ginger, and hot peppers all seem to have an effect on this substance.

Useful Combinations

As useful as turmeric is for so many conditions, it's a little tricky to get enough of it where the body needs it most. This is because the body tends to metabolize turmeric quickly, meaning it uses it all up. Herbalists and pharmacologists have found a few ways around this.

Black pepper. One of the chemicals in ordinary black pepper, piperine, seems to improve the bioavailability of turmeric. In fact, researchers at St. John's Medical College in Bangalore, India, found that combining turmeric with black pepper may significantly increase the body's ability to use it.

The combination of black pepper and turmeric from your friendly spice rack is perfect for people who are on a budget—and these days, I'd say that's just about everyone. Go to an Indian grocery store and choose the yellowest variety of turmeric you can find. I think you can safely guess that the yellower it is, the more curcumin it contains. A one-pound bag should cost between $3 and $5, a lot cheaper than what you'll pay for brand-name versions of turmeric, which usually have a hefty price of $3 for just a few grams. While you're there, get an ounce of fresh black peppercorns. Grind the peppercorns into powder and mix it with the turmeric. You've just created a 10-month supply of anti-inflammatory medicine for around $5.

Take half a teaspoon of the mixture three times a day. Some people mix it in chicken or tomato soup. If your tastebuds can stand it, you can swirl the mixture in a glass of water and slug it down.

For external use, this mixture works great as a poultice on sore joints—if you don't mind that your skin will turn a little yellow. To make the poultice, mix a little of the blend with warm castor oil and soak a cloth in it. Wrap the cloth around the sore joint, then wrap that with plastic wrap. Leave the poultice in place for about 40 minutes.

Isoflavonoids. For preventing cancer, you can't do better than mixing turmeric with foods that contain large amounts of isoflavonoids, some of which have powerful anti-cancer effects. In fact, some breast cancer researchers believe a combination of curcumin and isoflavonoids might be the most potent inhibitor of human breast tumor cells. You can get a lot of isoflavonoids in dried beans and peas, soy, kudzu, and licorice. Curried lentil or bean soups top my list here.

Pineapple. This fragrant tropical fruit is rich in a compound called bromelain. Some experts believe that turmeric and bromelain mixed together have a singularly powerful effect. I recommend slicing or dicing a cup or two of pineapple and larding it liberally with ginger and tumeric. I would also add a little papaya because it tastes great with pineapple. You can eat the spiced fruit as often as you want, keeping in mind that the acids in pineapple can be hard on the mouth when you eat too much.

People who enjoy the convenience of supplements can get similar effects by taking both curcumin and bromelain in capsule form. The recommended dose is 250 milligrams of bromelain and 250 to 500 milligrams of curcumin taken three times a day between meals. This is probably effective, but I always recommend using whole foods whenever possible.

Caution: Contraindications, Interactions, and Side Effects

I once thought it hard to imagine that anyone would eat enough turmeric to experience significant side effects, but I've since heard from one cancer survivor who had trouble taking it in food and finds the standardized capsules much easier.

Gastrointestinal problems. There are some suggestions in medical literature that people with gastrointestinal problems such as gallstones, stomach ulcers, hyperacidity, or bile duct obstructions shouldn't eat large amounts of turmeric, although I suspect these cautions may have been overstated. The German E Commission (a panel of experts roughly equivalent to the U.S. Food and Drug Administration) has advised against turmeric only for those people with biliary obstruction.

Apart from this, there's some evidence that having too much turmeric may cause stomach irritation in people who are sensitive to it. The irritation may be merely annoying, or it could lead to ulcers in supersensitive people.

Cell damage alert. Eating very large amounts of turmeric could potentially damage white and red blood cells. As a practical matter, however, there is little likelihood that anyone would ever ingest enough to make this happen.

Index

Boldface page references indicate illustrations. Underscored references indicate boxed text.

Garlic *(continued)*
for treating *(continued)*
lead poisoning, <u>112</u>
ulcers, peptic, <u>120</u>
wounds and sores, <u>37</u>
turmeric with, 127–28
vampire bats and, <u>111</u>
Gas, 73
Gastrointestinal problems, 246.
See also specific types
Genes, 6–7
Genitourinary problems, 175
Gilroy Garlic Festival, <u>117</u>
Ginger, 77–78, 182, 238,
<u>242–43</u>
Ginkgo, **129**
allergy and, 135, 142–43
"bleeding time" test and,
142
Chinese use of, <u>134</u>
combinations with, 141–42
components of, <u>133</u>
dosages of, 140–41
drug interactions with, 142
European sales of, <u>130</u>
horse chestnut with, 166
medicinal power of, general,
12, 129–32
new research on, <u>131</u>
recipe using, <u>141</u>
safety issues, 142
species of, 130–31
synthesis of, first, <u>136</u>
for treating
allergies, 135
altitude sickness, 135

Alzheimer's disease, 129,
132, 135–36
asthma, 136
capillaries, broken, 137
cellulite, <u>131</u>
eczema, 137
impotence, 137
intermittent claudication,
137–38, <u>139</u>
macular degeneration, 138
memory problems, 132,
134–35
migraines, 138–39
peripheral occlusive arterial
disease, <u>139</u>
radiation sickness, <u>131</u>
Raynaud's disease,
139–40
sickle cell anemia, <u>131</u>
tinnitus, 140
varicose veins, 137
Ginkgolides, 136, 139
Ginkgo tree, <u>142</u>
GLA. *See* Gamma-linolenic
acid
Glaucoma, 57, 59–60
Goldenseal, <u>43</u>, 95
Gout, <u>59</u>, 67, <u>68–71</u>, 76–77
Grapefruit juice, avoiding use
with herbs, 51
Growing herbs, <u>42–43</u>

H
Hair loss and regrowth, <u>165</u>,
225–26, 231–32

Hawthorn, **145**
  Chinese use of, <u>153</u>
  combinations with, 152–53
  depression and, 154
  dosages of, 21, 152
  drug interactions with,
    154–55
  garlic with, 127
  historical perspective of,
    <u>153</u>
  medicinal power of, general,
    12–13, 145–48
  Native American use of,
    <u>153</u>
  as ornamental, <u>146</u>
  pregnancy and, 154
  safety issues, 154–55
  species of, 146–47
  for treating
    angina pectoris, 148–49
    arrhythmia, 149, <u>155</u>
    atherosclerosis, 149–50
    cardiovascular insufficiency,
      150
    dyspnea, 150
    edema, 150
    heart problems, 145–50,
      <u>148</u>, <u>151</u>
    high cholesterol, 150–51
    hypertension, 150
HDL, 118
Headaches, 106, 138–39,
  176
Health insurance, 2–3
Health problems, 2–3. *See also
  specific types*

Heart problems. *See also specific
  types*
  celery seed and, 73–74
  garlic and, 78, 118–19
  hawthorn and, 145–50, <u>148</u>,
    <u>151</u>
  turmeric and, 240
Hemorrhoids, 160–61
Hepatitis, <u>89</u>, 190–91, <u>192</u>
Hepatopulmonary syndrome
  (HPS), <u>120</u>
Herbs. *See also specific types*
  aging and, 1, 17, 20
  allergic reaction to, 51
  antioxidants and, <u>10–11</u>
  brands of, 31–32, 46–47
  breastfeeding and, <u>19–20</u>
  buying, 31, 39–41, 44–48
  children and, 17, <u>19–20</u>
  combinations with, 22–23
  cost of, <u>4</u>, 32, 47
  dosages of, 21–22, 40, 50
  drying, <u>43–45</u>
  Duke's recommended dozen,
    9–13, 16–17
  effectiveness of, 32
  food farmacy approach and,
    <u>26–28</u>, <u>34–37</u>
  forms of, <u>34–37</u>, 38–39
  genes and, 6–7
  grapefruit juice with,
    avoiding, 51
  growing, <u>42–43</u>
  holistic approach and, 33,
    38
  improvements in, 7–8

M

Macular degeneration, 55, 57, 60–61, 138
MAOIs. *See* Monoamine oxidase inhibitors
Mayapple, 8
Memory problems, 132, 134–35
Menopause, 211
Migraines, 138–39
Milk thistle, 185
  combinations with, 195–98
  dosages of, 21, 194–95
  echinacea with, 196–98
  European research on, 189
  historical perspective of, 186
  medicinal power of, general, 13, 16, 185–90
  new research on, 192–93
  safety issues, 198
  sunflower seed oil and, 185
  for treating
    alcoholism, 190
    cirrhosis, 190
    hepatitis, 190–91
    liver problems, 185, 188–91
    pollution, 191
Minerals, 8–9. *See also specific types*
Monoamine-oxidase inhibitors (MAOIs), 206, 207, 210–11, 214
Mood enhancement, 209, 214
Morning sickness, 243
Motion sickness, 243
Mouth problems, 177

MS, 102–3
Multiple-herb formulas, 41, 44
Multiple sclerosis (MS), 102–3
Mushroom poisoning, 193

N

Neurotransmitters, 204
Niacin, 51
Niacin flush, 51
Night vision problems, 56, 57, 61
Nonsteroidal anti-inflammatory drugs (NSAIDs), 4
Nutritional medicine, 8–9

O

Obesity, 210
Oligomeric proanthocyanidins (OPCs), 146, 148, 149, 152
Onion, 122–24, 127–28
OPCs. *See* Oligomeric proanthocyanidins
Oregano, 78
Oxidation, 10–11, 78

P

PAF, 135–36
Pansies, 167–68
Parkinson's disease, 210–11
Passionflower, 180
Perimenopause, 211

Smoking cessation, 210
Spider veins, 162, 164
Sports injuries, 165
SSRI. *See* Selective serotonin
    reuptake inhibitor
Stinging nettle, 106, 231
Stomach problems, 128
Stores and clerks, herbal,
    47–48
Storing dried herbs, 45
Stress reduction, 23, 172–74,
    179–81, 180
Sulfur, 113
Sun-damaged skin, 88
Sunflower seeds and oil, 104,
    188
Sunscreen, 212, 214
Supplements, 8–9, 22, 25,
    28–29, 45

T

Teas, 34–35
Tegra, 119
Terpenes, 133
Throat disorders, 94
Tinctures, 35–36, 38–39
Tinnitus, 140
Tomato, 231
Toxicity, 66, 143
Transurethral resection of the
    prostate (TURP), 225
Tryptophan, 101, 104, 105
Turmeric, 235
    anti-inflammatory benefits of,
    235–37, 237, 240–41

celery seed with, 77
color of, 236
combinations with, 244–45
dosages of, 21, 241, 244
garlic with, 127–28
medicinal power of, general,
    16–17, 235–36
metabolism of, 244
poultices, 37, 241, 244
recipe using, 240
safety issues, 245–46
saffron and, 236
for treating
    arthritis, 235–36
    athlete's foot, 237
    heart problems, 240
    HIV, 240
    liver problems, 240
    skin problems, 241
    wounds and sores, 37,
    241
TURP, 225

U

Ulcers, peptic, 120
Unipolar depressions, 206
Uric acid, 67
Urinary tract infections, 58–59

V

Valerian, 180–81
Varicose veins, 137, 159,
    161–63, 163, 164
Venereal warts, 8

Violets, 167–68
Viral disorders, 8
Vitamins, 8–9. *See also specific types*
Vitamin C, 66
Vitamin E, 58

Wounds and sores, 37, 92–94, 204, 212, 241
Wrinkles, 165

Y

Yeast infections, 89

W

Walnuts, 153–54
Willow bark, 181
Witch hazel, 168

Z

Zinc, 95
Zoloft, 16, 206–7, 214–15